OXFORD MEDICAL PUBLICATIONS

Searching for Causes of Work-Related Diseases

Searching for Causes of Work-Related Diseases

An Introduction to Epidemiology at the Work Site

JØRN OLSEN
University of Aarhus, Denmark

FRANCO MERLETTI
University of Turin, Italy

DAVID SNASHALL
St. Thomas's Hospital, University of London

and

KAREL VUYLSTEEK
University of Gent, Belgium

OXFORD NEW YORK TOKYO
OXFORD UNIVERSITY PRESS

This book has been printed digitally and produced in a standard specification in order to ensure its continuing availability

OXFORD
UNIVERSITY PRESS

Great Clarendon Street, Oxford OX2 6DP

Oxford University Press is a department of the University of Oxford.
It furthers the University's objective of excellence in research, scholarship,
and education by publishing worldwide in

Oxford New York

Auckland   Cape Town   Dar es Salaam   Hong Kong   Karachi
Kuala Lumpur   Madrid   Melbourne   Mexico City   Nairobi
New Delhi   Shanghai   Taipei   Toronto
With offices in
Argentina   Austria   Brazil   Chile   Czech Republic   France   Greece
Guatemala   Hungary   Italy   Japan   South Korea   Poland   Portugal
Singapore   Switzerland   Thailand   Turkey   Ukraine   Vietnam

Oxford is a registered trade mark of Oxford University Press
in the UK and in certain other countries

Published in the United States
by Oxford University Press Inc., New York

© ECSC-EEC-EAEC Brussels-Luxembourg 1991

The moral rights of the author have been asserted

Database right Oxford University Press (maker)

Reprinted 2011

ISBN 978-0-19-261819-1

Printed and bound in Great Britain by CPI Antony Rowe,
Chippenham and Eastbourne

Foreword

W.W. Holland, St. Thomas's Hospital, University of London

The Panel for Epidemiology and Social Medicine in the European Community represents the academic societies working in this field within the Community. It attempts to advise the Commission on areas within its sphere of competence and reacts to Commission requests for advice. A further major function of the Panel is the identification of areas where education and instruction are required and the provision of the necessary education and instruction.

The investigation of occupational hazards is a concern for all Community countries. This short book is an outstanding description of the ways in which health hazards can be investigated using epidemiological techniques, how these can be carried out, and what the necessary prerequisites are to drawing conclusions from such studies.

The work has been undertaken by a number of individuals from each of the Community countries. It demonstrates how scientists can collaborate to produce a manual which should prove of great benefit to those concerned with the management of industry or investigation of outbreaks or possible causes of hazard and damage as a result of the work place. I am grateful to the members of the editorial board for their production of this highly readable and instructive work.

Preface

The European Community has committed itself to work for the 'Health for All' strategy developed by the Work Health Organization. In that programme specific targets are suggested to be reached before the year 2000. Target 25 specifies that, by 1995, people of the European region should be effectively protected against work-related health risks. Epidemiological skills are now needed to obtain the knowledge essential to making this goal achievable.

As most people spend a large part of their lives at the work place, and as some workers may be at risk of being exposed to harmful substances at quite high levels, it seems reasonable that workers' protection should have a high priority. Studies will help to identify causes of occupational diseases, and the outcome of such investigations should be applied when the effects of protective actions are evaluated. Research into causes and methods of evaluation of results usually have to be based on epidemiological principles.

There are many such problems compared with the number of professional researchers, therefore some research principles should be familiar to everyone concerned with workers' health—the occupational physician, the occupational health nurse, the shop steward, the worker himself. This book is written for people engaged in health promotion at the work site who have no formal training in epidemiology. Originally, we had occupational health nurses in mind but hope that many others will benefit from reading this book. It is not intended to create professional epidemiologists but to improve and sharpen abilities to solve health problems at the work site. We hope that, having read the book, you will know more about what you can do when a work-related health problem arises, and when to call on a professional epidemiologist for help.

Improving workers' health is an important step towards improving the health of the population at large and understanding the occupational causes of diseases will help us to improve our environment and provide better and safer living conditions for us all.

HOW TO USE THIS BOOK

This is not a textbook of epidemiology. There are several textbooks available and you should consult one of these if you have ambitions to make epidemiology a part of your daily work. This book is an appetizer, a gentle introduction to a subject which is often considered to be complicated and abstract.

People engaged in occupational medicine are periodically faced with a problem of ill-health amongst their work force: a number of workers within a given time period have become ill. Is this related to the work they do?

This first part is about the fundamental concepts of how to seek information about occupational causes of diseases. Part two works through some typical examples of epidemiological studies in the work place. Similar problem-solving principles are applied to problems which did actually occur at the work site and which were solved or at least properly described. Do you agree that initial analysis at the work site level helped in the decision to explore the problems further?

The glossary will be useful when reading the increasing volume of literature on epidemiology which often uses technical words. Try to learn the vocabulary so that the technicalities are easier to understand. The concepts are not difficult and can be worked with at a basic level. Should aspects of the problems become too complicated, you will need help from experienced epidemiologists. However, if you understand the basic principles you will be much better suited to be a co-worker and both parties will benefit.

Aarhus   J.O.
June 1990   F.M.
                                              D.S.
                                              K.V.

Acknowledgements

This project was supported by the Commission of the European Communities, Contract 86/036. We are most grateful to Walter Holland and to all members of the Panel for Social Medicine and Epidemiology in the European Economic Communities for useful discussions, encouragement, and support.

We would like to thank a number of people for useful comments and criticism on early drafts of the book. As authors we are responsible for the content of the book. However, we are particularly grateful to Guy De Backer, Marco Biocca, Giuseppe Costa, Alan Dalton, Tony Fletcher, John Fox, Elsebeth Lynge, Walter Holland, Svend Sabroe, Seb Schmoller, Benedetto Terracini, and Michel Van Hoorne.

Contents

Introduction

WHAT IS EPIDEMIOLOGY?

Several definitions of epidemiology have been suggested. The simplest is that epidemiology is the study of the occurrence of disease or other health-related characteristics in human populations. Quite often epidemiologists study not only the frequency of disease but why the frequency differs in different groups of people. Diseases do not occur at random; they have causes, quite often man-made causes, which are avoidable. Thus, many diseases may be prevented if the causes are known.

Many people are affected by the occurrence of diseases and their causes. Epidemiology is, therefore, not a discipline used only by professional researchers. The principles of epidemiological research are used by many people who do not even consider themselves epidemiologists. Modern epidemiology is a broad discipline which deals with determinants or risk indicators of a variety of health-related events in human populations. Much of our present knowledge in occupational medicine is drawn from epidemiological studies.

Many epidemiological studies in the field of occupational health start with the experience of the workers themselves. Often the workers—those exposed—knew that something was wrong long before this was confirmed by research. Occupational epidemiology can be thought of as a way of 'making sense' of workers' experience, of collecting and grouping the data in a proper way, and allowing inferences to be made on the occupational causes of their ill-health. Furthermore, the workers themselves, their representatives, and the people in charge of workers' health are the most appropriate persons to interpret the data which are collected. They should always be active participants in any investigation conducted at the work place. Only their direct involvement will guarantee that the work place will remain safe after the researchers have left. The aim of any study is the use of the results in the prevention of disease and the success of this depends to a large extent on ensuring that the 'exposed' participate in obtaining and interpreting the results.

WHERE ARE THE PROBLEMS? WHO WILL SOLVE THEM?

Workers and people in charge of workers' health, whether health professionals or not, may one day be confronted with problems such as:

- A number of truck drivers complain of low back pain. Could this be caused by new cabin seats?
- Six welders have now been treated for laryngeal cancer. Could this be the result of exposure to welding fumes?
- Since video-display terminals were introduced into the office, four women have had miscarriages. Could there be a connection?
- A new chemical is used by the dry-cleaners. Is it safe for the people in contact with this chemical?

As questions of this type arise some of the preliminary investigations have to be conducted by the people engaged in health at the work site, be it the workers themselves, shop stewards, or the occupational health nurse. The history of occupational medicine shows clearly that the observations of the workers themselves are of importance. If workers think that they have a health problem related to their work, this should be investigated because they have often been right, and the recognition has sometimes come too late. The saying 'as mad as a hatter', for example, exemplifies the fact that it was common knowledge that felt-hat workers were exposed to chemicals which caused psychological illness. Later, epidemiologists and toxicologists found that the culprit was mercury—a compound of which was used in the felting process. Clearly this type of information is needed urgently so that processes can be modified before more workers are made ill. However, the information alone is not sufficient. The first paper on mercurialism in hatters was published in 1860 but the hatters' occupational disease was not curbed until 1941 when mercury became needed for war production (Wedeen 1989). This historical fact is an important reason for involving workers more directly in occupational epidemiology.

Many studies start at the work site and important parts of the research work cannot take place anywhere else. Grass-roots epidemiology has the advantage that not only health professionals but all those involved will realize the importance of keeping records, pay-rolls, exposure data, etc. Key materials often lack in an investigation because there are inadequate exposure registers to match the registers of deaths and diseases. Research would be much aided if there was access to data on workers' past exposure. If working with a certain epoxy glue did cause cancer, that information would emerge immediately if all workers exposed to that glue in the previous 10–30 years could be identified.

In occupational health, any delay in identifying a problem can translate itself into an illness or even death. This book will prove useful when the question is asked: 'could this cluster of disease be caused by the work we do, or the work we have done?' We recommend that the basic principles of problem solving should be applied to the daily work of maintaining workers health:

(1) Define the health problem:
    (a) Does it exist?
    (b) What is the nature of the problem?
    (c) What are the possible explanations?
    (d) What are the possible consequences?
    (e) How important is the problem?

(2) Define the goal:
    (a) If the nature of the problem is known, describe what to do and set a goal for the outcome of this process;
    (b) If the nature of the problem is not known, set up a study plan for further investigation.

(3) Define the target group.

(4) Define the actions to be taken.

(5) Was the action plan followed?

(6) Measure the effect.

(7) Was the goal achieved? If not start all over again.

AIM AND SOURCES OF DATA

All of us, whether occupational health professionals, employees, captains of industry, or epidemiologists, if we are to fulfil our role in preventive health, need to ask questions. We need to be suspicious about diseases and injuries which occur to working people and about processes and substances, both old and new, which are used at work. We must also question peoples' habits, their diets, their hobbies, and their motives for behaving in a particular way at work or in volunteering that they are suffering from a particular disease. Most of the links between work and disease have started with an observation by somebody who was being suspicious or merely curious and there is no doubt that without this attitude little progress would be made. This means that a lot of problems of occupational health can be distinguished from the myriad claims of journalists and others who delight in every new association found between radiation and leukaemia, lead and child development, or fibre-glass and lung disease.

Whether the suspicion is that of a possible cluster of diseases such as cancer or the introduction of a new chemical or a new work process, the occupational health professional is in the best position to gather the relevant facts. Without good quality basic facts any number of fine epidemiologists and powerful computers are unimportant.

Suppose, to take the simplest kind of example, you noticed there is a greater than usual absence from work amongst the employees of a chicken-processing factory and the rumour is that they are all suffering from sore wrists due to the introduction of a new packaging machine which increases the number of chickens being processed every day. There may of course be 'political' objections to anyone trying to investigate this kind of outbreak and the best thing, if possible, is to bring the subject up at a health and safety meeting attended by representatives of management and unions. If there is no such formal structure then a direct approach to a local trades union official is probably the answer. The management themselves might wish some investigation to be made into the matter. If none of these routes is possible for local reasons then some support for an investigation and some advice on how to go about it can be obtained from the local branch of the

Health and Safety Executive. They may refer the enquiry to an employment medical adviser who is usually a doctor experienced in disentangling such problems. Preparing the ground and obtaining permission to begin which is agreed by as many representatives as possible is an essential first step which you can then follow by asking some simple questions. You will want to know the size, age range and sex of the work force. In the absence of a finance department or a personnel department you may simply have to piece the information together as best you can so that the number of persons off work and the amount of time for which they have been off work can be computed. There will undoubtedly be records available on these aspects held either centrally or at shop-floor manager level. Then the diagnosis which has probably been decided upon either by the employees themselves, their general practitioners, or specialists needs to be checked. The diagnosis should be confirmed by a doctor for reasons of confidentiality and because many different names may be given to this condition, usually termed 'repetitive strain injury' (RSI). In this way you can build-up a picture of the type of injury, the number of people who have it and for how long they have had it. The other part of the cause-and-effect equation is to look at what the people who have the injury do as part of their work and what the rest of the people who do not have the injury do as part of their work. Certain people will know when the new processes for chicken-packing were brought in and others will know the rate of injury. With all this information about the individuals, their medical condition, and the processes which might have caused this condition collected as accurately as possible from the various sources mentioned, a case can be made as described elsewhere (p. 47) in this book and your suspicions of the cause of the problem confirmed or squashed. This is a simple example which can be settled at the local level without the need for much professional help and given a co-operative management and work force, the success of any remedial measures can be monitored over the ensuing months by simply measuring sickness absence.

The problem may involve a more serious or long-standing disease, or one which has resulted in a number of people dying. This presents a much greater problem in collecting accurate information about the diseased people. Local information might be helpful from, for example company pension records, trades union pension records, or occupational health records held by the company. Cases of certain diseases which are rare such as leukaemia in a particular area have even been traced by meticulously working through obituaries in local newspapers and checking these against death certificates. Local doctors may help to complete the picture and there may be lists of people who used to work in the company and who receive newsletters etc. These amateur detective techniques are all useful in building up a crude picture of a suspiciously high disease rate. It is difficult for the non-professional to go beyond this crude fact finding. However, if you want to know more about particular kinds of disease and their possible relationship to working conditions, there are various institutions which can often help. For a specific industry there is often a body of information held by the appropriate trades federation or trades union or society of interested members from whom you can get some ideas. Alternatively, a medical library, medical school, department of community health or environmental health, or the Health and Safety Executive may be able to help. These institutions can arrange computer searches which may give you some of the information you are looking for.

One of the most satisfactory ways of finding out the cause of death is from the death certificate. In Britain (although this is not the case in all countries, including some European ones) this is not a private document. Relatives of the deceased may have a copy of the death certificate as may personnel departments, medical departments, or pension departments of certain companies. Death certificates may also be obtained from the Office of Population Census and Surveys (OPCS), a service which has to be paid for. Even though they are the most accurate record of disease leading to death that we are likely to have they are unfortunately not always as accurate as one would like and are sometimes difficult to interpret—you may need a doctor or epidemiologist to do this for you. In the case of a prolonged disease you will not be interested only in those people who have died from the disease, but also those who have suffered from it without dying or before dying from it. This information is more difficult to obtain, but there are records available in hospitals, and certain registers of disease (such as cancer) are kept available usually only to professional researchers or epidemiologists. These lists are of course extremely valuable and can help to substantiate your crude measures of disease. If you think that a particular disease in your particular study population in a factory for example is higher or lower than 'normal' you will need to know what the 'normal' disease incidence is in, for example, the general population or perhaps a population of similar workers in another factory. This kind of information on disease rates is also available from OPCS.

The work place

If it is intended to try to make a link between diseases or accidents and substances or processes then knowledge about the work place must be gleaned as accurately as possible. Again it is important to have the backing of a trade union or management before embarking on this kind of investigation and, depending on the size .of the organization in question, information on these aspects of the work will come from different areas. Information on processes may come from trade federations or from organizations which represent whole industries e.g. glass-making, ceramics etc. Information on the factory in question is more likely to come from personnel departments, finance departments (often a useful guide to how many people there are, and when they started and finished). Engineering and works departments in certain industries keep technical data and in some factories records on individual exposure have been kept for many years. However, the methods for collecting exposure information have varied greatly over the years and not all the information is of good quality. Exposure may be recorded as the concentration in air of a chemical in a particular laboratory or information taken from personal sampling instruments or regular biological tests on the workers themselves. There is statutory monitoring of some individuals, for example deep-sea divers, workers with ionizing radiation, lead, and asbestos and these records are kept by the Health and Safety Executive. A rough estimate of exposure can often be made by looking at the person's job title.

In a cement factory for instance, a packer is more likely to be exposed than a lorry driver. There are new EEC regulations and new regulations in the UK (Control of Substances Hazardous to Health) which specify the way in which certain processes and substances have to be monitored and assessed, and the way in which workers exposure to such substances should be controlled.

This information has to be kept for 50 years and so will be a useful source of records for the future. In many industries exposure records may be missing for a variety of reasons, for example the industry may have ceased to exist and its records may have been lost or destroyed. It is worth having a search for them in case they have only been mislaid. Information on substances used at the work place can often be obtained from a supplies department or a safety department, if one exists. All substances used in industry now have to be labelled properly, and there is a hazard sheet available from the manufacturers on each one. This has not always been the case. General information on the toxicity of substances and other relevant literature may be available from the research departments of specific industries, for example oil industry, fertilizer industry. There may be health records on employees which list previous occupations and exposures and give an idea of current or past exposures in the present employment.

Much of the basic information on diseases, processes, and substances can be collected by the non-professional at the work place or the occupational health professional. In the simpler cases involving a small number of people the methods described in this book will enable you to come to a fair conclusion on the likelihood of disease and exposure being linked. However, at a certain point the amateur detective technique must give way to more powerful and sophisticated methods which is where the epidemiologists and statisticians come in to their own. Call them in sooner rather than later, because even if they do not become involved at once they will be able to guide during your initial fact finding exercises.

Where do you find epidemiologists?

Epidemiologists trained in the disentanglement of occupational problems are few and far between. You may get some idea of one who is already interested in the particular problem you are investigating by asking the appropriate trades union or Health and Safety Executive to recommend somebody who could help. There are departments of occupational health throughout the UK and the rest of Europe who may be able to give epidemiological assistance. Departments of public health, community medicine or environmental medicine often contain such experts. Trades unions and other industrial organizations may have international links and you may find that even though nobody in your own country knows much about the particular subject you wish to follow up, there may be individuals in other countries who are interested and have already made some investigations.

The results

The conclusion to a formal study may be that there is an association between diseases observed and work processes, or that there is a possible or probable association needing more study. You may find that there is a definite association but it is difficult to define the way that the cause and effect operate, or you come across a clear-cut answer—the substance in question is found to cause the disease in question, and the process can be changed. It must be admitted that this kind of intellectually satisfying conclusion is exceptionally rare. Remember also that epidemiology is not always the best or final way to approach problems. Ergonomic research, toxicology, or animal experimentation may be valid alternatives.

PART I

Concepts of epidemiology

PROBLEMS AND POSSIBLE SOLUTIONS

An epidemiological study is often begun because a health problem exists and a solution is needed. The best solution would be to prevent diseases from occurring at the work place and sometimes that is possible. New chemicals or processes should ideally be tested before being used. However, no test based upon cells, bacteria, or animals will guarantee that the actual exposure is harmless for man. Chemical compounds can lead to very complex exposures and the damaging effect of this on health is difficult to predict or even document.

The second best solution to work site health problems is to try to detect them as soon as they appear; but to implement a monitoring system, good company records are needed. Even if the concern is not about a current problem, proper record systems should be maintained. These data may turn out to be the essential clues if something goes wrong.

- You will need these facts if an unexpectedly high number of health problems occurs.
- You will need good records, if a new—potentially harmful—work process is introduced.
- You have to think ahead of time. What could happen in the future?

Detectives on the job

In real life you are sometimes confronted with a cluster of diseases which might be related to an exposure at work. If a number of people become ill and that number exceeds what would normally be expected, you will want to know if the cause is related to the work environment. Looking for causes is similar to being a detective. Like a detective you want to know 'who did it' in order to stop further damage. Like a detective you have to work systematically, critically, and with an open mind. Some rules of thumb can be given and are presented in some detail in this book. Most of all you do not want to spend more time following false clues than is necessary.

Is there a problem?

Contracting a disease is always a problem for those involved but it is not necessarily a work-related problem. Only a few people go through life without having any diseases and in the end we all have to die, regardless of the work we do. More than one person in four contracts cancer during their lifetime. More than one male in three has a heart attack. Almost all will suffer from low back pain at some time. The mere existence of diseased workers does not imply that the problem is work-related. However, if there is an excess of sick workers, the cause may reside in the work place, especially if the rate of illness is much higher than would normally be expected.

Observed and expected

Comparing the observed number of cases with an expected number is one of the key techniques of epidemiology. When an epidemiologist hears that a number of people are sick, he or she will ask 'how many sick workers would you expect, had the employees *not* been exposed to anything at work?' In other words, what would be the number of sick people in a population of similar age, sex, and way of life?

A factory in Kentucky

At a factory in Kentucky, USA, four cases of a rare type of liver cancer were found within a short time among the 500 workers employed. This specific form of liver cancer occurs at a rate of 20–30 new cases per year in the entire US population of more than 200 million.

Clearly, four cases among 500 people is more than expected. In fact, it is so far above the expected number of cases, that one would first have to question the diagnoses. But the diagnoses were confirmed, the problem was real, and it turned out to be a problem of occupational origin, caused by intensive exposure to vinyl chloride monomer (the raw material used to make PVC).

When the number of diseased persons exceeds the expected number to this extent a reason should be found. The occurrence of disease varies from time to time and from population to population. It may reflect random or chance variation. Sometimes the occurrence even exceeds a level which makes chance variation a likely explanation but before any study starts we need to ask a few basic questions. We need to know something about the diseased.

Who, where, and when

Who are the diseased?

Epidemiology deals with groups of people rather than with individuals. This does not mean that individuals are neglected, but that cause-and-effect relationships are often impossible to study in a single individual. If you have an accident in a certain car, it does not necessarily follow that that particular car is more unsafe than any others. All types of cars have accidents now and then. But if a particular type of car has twice as many accidents as other types, then the production company and the drivers might have a problem.

Epidemiology compares the occurrence of diseases in two different groups of people. The number of new diseased individuals in a particular group of people depends upon the number of people in the group and the time period over which new cases are recorded. Thus the size of the group and the duration of the study is important. In epidemiology the occurrence of disease is described as a rate (an incidence rate) which is the number of new cases divided by the time during which each individual in the group has been under observation (from starting to record new cases until the end of our recording or until a person contracts the disease, *see* incidence rate in glossary).

An incidence rate depends upon the average risk of getting the disease during a particular time period. It is useful to know if one group has a risk which differs from a comparable group. The two groups are usually compared by dividing the incidence rate among the 'exposed' workers by the incidence rate among those not-exposed. This is a *relative* rate and it reflects how many times the risk among the exposed is higher than the risk among the not exposed. Were this calculated in the example from Kentucky it would show that the risk of liver cancer among the workers was many times higher than the risk of this cancer in the population at large. However, this partly reflects the fact that the risk among those not exposed is very low and when dividing any number by another number close to zero, the relative rate becomes very high. To some extent this could be misleading and hide the fact that still only a few (in absolute numbers) among the exposed get the disease. By presenting the risk among the workers compared with the population at large—not as a relative rate but as a rate difference—the rate among exposed minus the rate among the not-exposed, a more realistic idea of the excess risk is given.

Even though we are basically interested in comparing such rates in different groups we often start with something which at first seems to be quite different. We do not follow identified groups of people over time and calculate incidence rates, we simply start with the available information about the diseased.

Useful and necessary information

The epidemiologist usually collects information about groups of people, but basic information about individuals is also necessary. If you have a cluster of diseased, you should at least find out the following facts about them.

(1) Name or other personal identification.
(2) Date of birth, sex, and address.
(3) Dates and duration of all employments.
(4) Date of onset of disease/death.
(5) Diagnosis and the person or place where the diagnosis came from.
(6) Job history—as detailed and comprehensive as possible, especially concerning the timing of exposure.
(7) Important health-related life-style factors—for example smoking.

Having obtained these data you will be able to answer the first question: Who is ill? How many are ill? Where and when did they become ill? Often this simple, basic information can be very useful. In the Kentucky example it was very useful to know that liver cancer occurred at the beginning of the 1970s, in a factory producing polyvinyl chloride and among men who had been exposed to vinyl chloride for 10–20 years. As a detective you have some major suspicions but no proof which would stand up in court.

You need to know something about those who were affected by the disease, and those who were not. You need to know what is common and particular to the diseased. This is how a detective works and how clinicians make their deductions. Initially, it looks as if this information could not tell you anything about the risk among exposed compared with that among non-exposed, the number of not-exposed, nor the exact time of observation. You have to start off by collecting information on the diseased only. However, it turns out to be just one step in estimating relative rates among exposed versus non-exposed. To begin with the magnitude of the problem is of secondary importance; whether a problem exists or not, comes first.

Do the diseased have anything in common?

Like the detective who, faced with a number of similar crimes, would like to know if all the criminal acts were performed by the same person, the epidemiologist would like to know if a specific job or work process is responsible for all, or most of the damage. The epidemiologist looks for common exposures, common habits, common residence, etc. Most, if not all, diseases have several causes, and there may be more than one factor in common among the diseased. It might be that specific types of welding fume cause lung cancer, but so do a number of other exposures, tobacco smoke for example. Since some of the lung cancers we observe among workers are likely to have a different aetiology, no single exposure is likely to account for all the cases identified.

What distinguishes the diseased from the non-diseased?

The non-diseased may have had similar exposure to the diseased. All the diseased breathe air, eat, drink water and so on, and so do the non-diseased. This information is not very helpful in our effort to try to identify why the diseases occur in the first place. It would be much more informative to know about events which seem to be operating less frequently among the non-diseased.

If all the diseased, for example all those with the rare liver cancer, were exposed to vinyl chloride before the onset of the cancer and none of the rest were exposed, there would be a strong case to suspect the vinyl chloride. However, one would usually expect a proportion of the diseased not to have been exposed to the agent in question. Again the epidemiologist looks for exposures being more common among the diseased compared with the non-diseased (controls).

Comparison of exposure status and other background information between the diseased and the non-diseased is made in the case-control study—one of the tools often used by the work place detective, the local epidemiologist.

Men working with a worm-killing substance (1,2-dibromo-3-chloropropane, DBCP) recognized among themselves that few had recently fathered children. On investigation, 11 men were found to have very low sperm counts.

After recognition of this 'outbreak' of infertility, a case-control comparison was made among all workers who used DBCP. The cases, those with low sperm counts, were older and had worked for a longer time period with DBCP than had the controls. DBCP exposure seemed to be more frequent in the cases than in the non-cases.

Among 11 cases with low sperm counts the average exposure time to DBCP was 8.0 years. Among 11 controls with normal sperm counts the average exposure duration was 0.1 year (Whorton *et al.* 1977).

Why John and not Peter?

If you claim that, for example, a particular compound causes skin problems you have to answer questions like: John has never worked with that compound, yet he has the skin disease—and Peter has been using the compound for years, and he has no problem. How can the compound then be the cause? The same argument is applied to the case of life-long heavy smokers who never get lung cancer compared with non-smokers who do.

The reason for that is that few, if any, diseases have only one cause, and few causes, if any, can by themselves induce the disease. Therefore the compound in question is rarely the only cause of a given disease in a population. Often a set of causes are necessary to cause the disease. Peter might only be exposed to one, not all, of the causes—or he might be less susceptible to the disease. John might have acquired the disease from another set of causes.

The liver cancer case from Kentucky is unusual in that this particular type of liver cancer seems to have causes which occur with a very low frequency in the USA. In the factory area, vinyl chloride exposure must have been the most common cause. However, vinyl chloride exposure alone was not enough—not all those exposed to it developed cancer. Epidemiologists would say that vinyl chloride is not a sufficient cause; other exposures or perhaps genetic susceptibility must also be present for the disease to develop.

THE CASE-CONTROL STUDY

If a cluster—that is an unusual gathering of a specific disease, usually within a rather short time span—occurs at a given work site, this might of course be due to chance, but it could also be the result of a given set of exposures.

For the work-place detective facing an outbreak of disease, the chance explanation is the last conclusion to be reached. If all other explanations have been ruled out, chance might remain as the last likely explanation, but other possible explanations should be considered and excluded first. Or, in the words of that excellent detective, Sherlock Holmes 'When you have eliminated the impossible whatever remains, however improbable, must (may) be the truth'.

If a cluster of diseases occurs, start by making sure that the cluster is real—that the diseases did occur. Then start thinking of possible explanations for the clustering. For example, if a number of accidents occur at a particular crossroads, it could be a coincidence, but there are other possible explanations.

The recognition of a cluster of disease often comes by chance— often by a shrewd observation by a clinical doctor, (as for example, in the recognition of excess nasal cancer in furniture workers or the DBCP example) or even by astute journalists (such as was the case with childhood leukaemia cases in the vicinity of the Sellafield Nuclear Reprocessing Plant).

The study plan

Devising a plan for a case-control study requires some medical knowledge as well as the ability to think critically. In the schedule for the study you have to consider how to select cases and controls, what information you need, how to obtain it, and how the results are to be analysed. The purpose of the exercise is to narrow down the possible explanations for the unexpectedly high number of diseased. As a detective you are looking for the area on which to focus your attention to further your investigations. Did many of the diseased work with a new chemical compared with the non-diseased, for example?

As cases, you used the diseased which came to your attention, but first you should make sure they actually have the disease in question. Next you have to make sure you have all the diseased presenting over a given time period in the group you want to study. You should then think of how to define your study base (*see* glossary).

In the present context only a very general idea about how to conduct case-control studies is given. Large-scale case-control studies are for professional epidemiologists.

The original idea of the case-control study goes back many hundreds of years. If some exposure is more common to a number of circumstances that are associated with the disease and if that exposure is much more frequent for the diseased than for the non diseased, this factor may be one of the causes of the disease. Comparing diseased and not diseased in order to look for potential causes of disease is not a new idea at all. Only the principles for selecting diseased and controls are new, and these principles are largely guided by our desire to quantify the magnitude of association.

Some of the principles of the case-control technique can and should be applied during small scale investigations, whilst you are considering whether to call for extra assistance.

The main focus here is on a case-control study in a factory in which diseased and non-diseased workers, employed at the same factory, are compared with regard to previous exposures.

Study base

The study base comprises the group of people in which you take an interest. It is the population which supplies you with the cases you plan to include in your study.

- Are you interested only in people who worked at a particular plant at a given time?
- Are you interested in diseases occurring only among employed workers or do you want also to include retired workers?
- Are you interested in all workers, or only in workers of a given age or sex, or only workers with a given work history?

It depends upon the problem to be solved.

We know that we want to look for exposures which the diseased—the cases—might have in common, and then find out if these exposures are seen less frequently among the non-diseased—the controls. We do not want to make this comparison in a haphazard way, because the results will be unreliable. Some research principles must be followed.

One of these principles is to define the study base. It may be impossible to define the study base precisely. We want to make our comparisons within the group of people where the cases arose. That population is the base population for our study, but it may be impossible to tally and identify the population individual by individual, especially when there is a long period of time between the exposure and the disease. It is very important to have a precise idea of who is and who should be in the study base.

The case group

Having defined the study base, or at least identified some criteria for belonging to it, you should make an effort to identify all cases which occurred in that base population within the time period of interest. The case group could be all hospitalized patients with a given disease, all who complain about a number of symptoms, all who had a certain accident, and so on. It is often difficult to identify all those who fulfil the criteria set up for the case group, but the next task can be even more difficult. You have to identify a proper comparison group within the study base to compare with your cases. In some small scale studies, all remaining non-diseased individuals in the study base can serve as controls.

In the DBCP example, the study base was all men working in a given department of the plant. The case group was 11 workers with low sperm counts; the remaining 11 workers served as controls.

The control group

The control group (your comparison or reference group as it may also be called) should stem from the same study base, and one option is to take a random sample of all the people identified in that base population.

If you study diseases occurring among employed workers in, say the time period 1986 to 1988 and you identify 100 workers, you might randomly select, for example, 40 among the non-diseased as your comparison group. If possible you should also examine all 100 workers with regard to exposure. By studying exposure status among the diseased and comparing that with the exposure status of the total group of 100, you are also applying case-control techniques.

A case-control study is the retrospective recording of exposure and the disease. However, the exposure and disease onset is recorded in the proper time sequence. Assessment of exposure relates to the proper time period for potential causes of the disease, that is at least before the onset of the disease. In cancer studies it may be years before the disease, in accident research, seconds before the accident.

In the Kentucky example, the study base could be all those employed for at least five years in the particular factory within, for example 10 years before the liver cancer cases started to occur. A case-control study of this type might have shown that all liver cancer cases of that particular type were exposed to vinyl chloride compared with, say 40 per cent of all the remaining workers.

Defining the case group as all liver cancer patients from the study base might show that 50 per cent were exposed compared with the 40 per cent. A result of this kind would indicate that vinyl chloride is but one of the many causes of the liver cancer.

Another option is to match each case with a control. If you match on age and sex then you select the person in the study base with the same sex and with the closest possible date of birth as your control. It is of course possible to match on other things, such as income, place of residence, date of employment, etc. Matching is also used as a convenient way of selecting a control. For each person with low back pain within a certain factory, among the other workers the one with the closest possible birth date and same sex could be selected. By doing this the groups are matched according to age and sex.

If you match cases to controls according to what you believe may be other potential causes of the disease in question you should take this into consideration when analysing the data. Do not look at the frequency of exposure among all cases compared with the frequency among the not-exposed, which you would do without matching. Look instead at the frequency of pairs where the case was exposed and not the control and compare this with the number of pairs in which the case was exposed but not the control, by setting up a simple two by two table (Table 1(a) and 1(b)).

Table 1(a). Comparing exposure in an unmatched case-control study

Exposure	Cases	Controls
yes	a	b
no	c	d

$$OR = \frac{a/c}{b/d}$$

Table 1(b). Comparing exposure in a matched study of pairs of cases and controls

Control part of the pairs exposed	Case part of the pairs exposed	
	yes	no
yes	e	f
no	g	h

$$OR = \frac{g}{f}$$

In the two types of case-control studies (with or without matching) it is now possible to calculate the odds ratio (OR) which estimates the relative risk (RR) of the disease among the exposed compared to that of the non-exposed, in spite of the fact we have no data on all the people in the study base. (Refer to textbooks of epidemiology for details—only the simple way of doing this calculation is presented here. See further reading.)

If 40 workers start complaining of low back pain in a given factory in a given year. For each of these 40 people a matched person without low back pain is identified of the same sex and with the closest possible birthdate. 'Exposure' in this case could be operating a particular heavy machine. When the exposure of the 40 pairs of workers is analysed the results could be as shown in Table 1(c).

Table 1(c). Comparison of 40 pairs of workers

Control part of the pairs exposed	Case part of the pairs exposed		
	yes	no	all
yes	8	5	13
no	15	12	27

$$RR = \frac{15}{5} = 3$$

For 8 pairs both the case and the control were exposed, for 12 pairs none was exposed and these pairs gave no information on the risk of exposure. However, in 15 pairs only the ones with low back pain were exposed whereas in 5 pairs only the controls were exposed. These are the only pairs which can tell us about the risk of exposure and we estimate the incidence of low back pain among the exposed to be three times as high as for the not-exposed by simply dividing 15 by 5.

Unfortunately, there are no golden rules for selecting comparison groups in the case-control study. A proper definition of the study base and a random sample taken from the base as controls will often be suitable. However, there is one useful rule to apply when you are in doubt as to whether or not the controls stem from the same population as the case group. Think of what would have happened if one of the non-diseased had had the disease you are studying. Had this occurred the person should then have been in your case group; if not, the controls did not stem from the same study base. This might sound abstract but in practice it is not so difficult to understand. Take the case-control study of, say, DBCP exposure as a cause of infertility. For each control person try to think whether he would be in the case group had he fulfilled the entry criteria for that group. If so then both cases and controls come from the same study base.

In the example from Kentucky, one could also take interest in the association between vinyl chloride exposure and lung-cancer. Suppose that the exposure of lung-cancer patients from the factory was to be compared with the exposure among citizens randomly sampled from the population at large in the area. We would expect this exposure to be negligible, because they come from a different study base. The comparison is not valid. We are dealing with two different study bases for cases (only factory workers) and controls (all in the population). Only a few of the lung-cancer patients in the control group would become a member of the case group (only those employed at the factory).

The aim of the study should guide the selection of the study base. If you want to study whether working at the factory carries a high risk of lung-cancer, select the region of the factory as the study base. Include all lung-cancer patients from the region in the case group with a control group of people randomly selected from the same region (the same study base). If you want to study whether vinyl chloride exposure, or a specific work process, is associated with the disease, select the factory as the study base. All lung-cancer patients among employed people in the factory now enter the study base and their exposure experience is compared with a similar exposure experience from the remaining group of workers (or a sample from that group). Defining the study base is a matter of where to focus the attention.

We know that cabinet makers run a high risk of acquiring cancer of the nose but we do not exactly know why. Conducting a case-control study using as controls a sample of people in the region where we collected our nasal-cancer patients will not give more insight into the matter. It will only tell us what we already know, that cabinet makers have a high risk.

The problem is that we will have a number of cabinet makers

among the cases but only very few in the control group. When we compare occupational histories we have to compare cabinet makers with cabinet makers. A more efficient way to answer the question of *why* cabinet makers run a high risk (not *if* they run a high risk) is to restrict the study base to cabinet makers only.

Obtaining exposure information

Having selected the groups to study, the next challenge is to obtain objective and reliable information about the exposure of interest. Sometimes you can get this information directly by interviewing the cases and controls, but often you have to obtain information from other sources.

If your cases are people with low back pain, it is no good asking cases and controls to quantify the strain caused by the things they have to lift. A person with low back pain would find it strenuous to lift something of even moderate weight. Therefore the information from the cases is not comparable with the information from the workers with no low back pain. If you are interested in studying the importance of daily work-load and low back pain, you have to quantify the work-load in a much more objective way. On the other hand, if you just want to know if truck drivers have a higher risk of low back pain than any other workers, it might be sufficient to base the information upon personal interviews of cases and controls because they would all know their job title.

In the case-control study you start with a health problem and look for a solution. Even though you might be interested in specific exposures you seek information on other aspects as well. Diseases do not always have a single cause.

If you claim that welding fumes cause lung diseases, sooner or later you will be met with the question 'Didn't they get the lung disease because of smoking?' So in your case-control study you should look for that as well. Like a detective, you rule out other possible explanations and what remains must be the most likely explanation. You try to move as close to the truth as possible: you try to have a case that will stand up in court. If your cases smoke more than your controls, you will have to consider this later in the data analysis.

In the case-control study, disease has occurred and a causal explanation is sought. The study is set up to find out why the cases occurred. Sometimes it is possible to set up a study before the disease occurs and to follow exposed workers at risk of getting the disease we are looking for, i.e. a follow-up study.

If in doubt seek help. When the study is complete show the results to an epidemiologist in order to decide on further action. If you intend to involve other people in more than negligible data collection, or if you cannot finish your study within a short time span, seek help. Local detectives are helpful, if they know their own limitations and when to call for help. An initial study at the work site may, however, not only be helpful in identifying problems worthy of larger scale studies, but also in making sure that data will be available for such large scale studies.

THE FOLLOW-UP STUDY

A 'cause' looking for a disease

A cluster of disease often initiates a case-control study, but a clustering of diseases could easily escape notice. Good record keeping or registers are often very helpful; but experience, intuition, or chance may play a role. You have a problem and you need a solution. You have a group of diseases and you look for a cause. Epidemiological principles may also be applied if you have a new work process which might influence the health of the workers or a potential cause of harm and you need to know if it will influence the health of the workers. It is necessary to find out whether a particular exposure damages workers' health.

In this case you have an exposure—a number of people are exposed. The problem is: does it damage the workers' health?

In the Kentucky example, it would have been possible to identify a group of workers exposed to vinyl chloride and study new diseases occurring in the study period: a control group, which might be non-exposed workers from the same factory would be needed.

Again define your potential problem, ask who, where, when. This time you do not start with a health problem which needs an explanation. You start out with an exposure which might be harmful. In this case you should know as much as possible about the exposure. What chemicals? What levels? What happens in the work process? Are there peak exposures? Is anything known about their toxicology? Look up the existing literature.

Record factors 1,2,3,6, and 7 on p. 14 for all the exposed (and for the comparison group) and be sure to record the main medically verified health problems they may have had before starting the work process. The exposure may cause harm, but cannot be responsible for diseases that occurred before the exposure started. You can be sure someone will ask if the disease is 'new' when you claim that backache was caused by heavy lifting.

A detective shadowing a suspect does not know what crime to expect (if any) but sometimes there might be a clue from the criminal record. This may make it clear that a bank robbery is much more likely to be perpetrated than a sex offence. Previous experience of the exposure in question may point more towards specific diseases and the study should be prepared in such a way that these diseases are surveyed. Some knowledge of pathophysiology comes in useful here because it is quite possible that, for example, exposure to noise may cause diseases other than hearing loss. Noisy conditions might well predispose to a raised accident rate, but are unlikely to contribute to the incidence of gout.

The ongoing follow-up study

The detective who follows the suspect and finally catches him in the act has a strong case. He might have spent a lot of time waiting for something to happen, but when it happens he is ready for it. Conceptually, this is more satisfactory than being confronted with a crime and having to dig up the evidence.

However, the follow-up study is time-consuming. You need to be patient, but such study is in itself simpler than a case-control study: you identify a number of exposed, you select a comparison group of non-exposed, and wait.

If you have equal sized groups of exposed and non-exposed (controls), you simply want to see if you have more diseased among the exposed compared with the controls during the same follow-up time. If the groups are of unequal size or if you have a different follow-up time, you must take that into consideration when making the comparison (see the section on incidence and prevalence), Table 2.

Table 2. The simplest presentation of follow-up study results

Exposure	Diseased	All	Observation time
+	a	n_+	t_+
−	c	n_-	t_-

Relative risk $= \dfrac{a/n_+}{c/n_-}$

Rate ratio $= \dfrac{a/t_+}{c/t_-}$

'All' in the table indicates those who entered the exposure study group, (n_+), or the non-exposed group (n_-) at the time of the study. The observation time is the time during which these groups have been under observation, i.e. the time from the beginning of the study (not necessarily the same as the beginning of exposure) to its end, or until the disease develops during the study period. If ten people are followed for one year and one of these develops the disease in the middle of that year, the observation time is 9y + 0.5y = 9.5 years (see glossary for details). If all were followed throughout the follow-up time, the relative risk indicates the proportion of diseased in the time period divided by the same proportion amongst the non-diseased. The rate ratio indicates the incidence rate amongst the exposed divided by the incidence rate amongst non-exposed. In most cases, when the selected groups can be followed throughout the study period the relative risk and the rate ratio will be very similar.

Selecting exposed and non-exposed

In the follow-up study, you also start by defining a study base. This is identified person by person. You identify a group of people at risk of the diseases you want to associate with the exposure.

In the case-control study you had to identify your study base back in time. You had—in the abstract—to identify the group of people in which the cases arose. In the follow-up study, you identify the study base yourself. Selecting people at risk implies they do not have the disease when the observation starts and their risk of getting the disease within the study period is more than zero. You are wasting your time if you follow male welders in order to see if welding fumes cause cervical cancer. Similarly, you do not study spontaneous abortions in women above the age of 45 years; you select women who are likely to become pregnant. It is not essential that you identify all exposed individuals, but it is important that the group of non exposed you compare with the exposed has a similar risk of getting the disease at the time of onset of the exposure.

A follow-up study on hearing loss could, for example, be made in a population with one group of workers being exposed to a noisy engine, and the others not so. Both cohorts will usually be followed for a number of years.

The study base is thus a group of exposed and a group of non-exposed from amongst the workers. Alternatively all the workers of a factory (exposed) and the general population (non-exposed) are compared and a standardized mortality ratio (*see* glossary) is computed. In such a case a number of problems of interpretation can arise.

Healthy worker selection

It is rarely a good idea to compare mortality among full-time employed workers with the mortality of the general population. Being in full-time employment implies a level of good health, and a group of full-time employed workers will include only a few people with chronic diseases. On the other hand, the total population will also include the people who—for health reasons— cannot work, and most of these people have a higher than average mortality. For this reason alone, you might find a lower mortality among the exposed compared with the population in general, even when the exposure does not influence morbidity and mortality. The comparison is biased, and the results say more about the health status of full-time workers than of the effect of exposure. In the literature you will often find this low mortality among the exposed referred to as the 'healthy worker effect'.

The 'healthy worker effect' is often the result of two different types of selection. In the first place, people with ill-health often avoid a job which they think will not suit their particular health problem—sometimes even a formal pre-placement medical exam- ination has to be passed. Secondly, ill-health might influence length of employment in a particular job. If health plays a role at the time of employment or for the 'survival' in the job this should be taken into consideration.

It is well known that some occupations have a lower mortality rate than that of the population at large. For instance some occupational groups such as Finnish foundry and granite workers or American steel, rubber, and chemical workers, have mortality rates 10–20 per cent less than the population average. This is explained by 'healthy worker selection'.

Follow-up time

The cause-effect mechanism takes place over time. However, the disease rarely follows immediately after the beginning of exposure. Usually it takes time, often years, for a disease to emerge. Many occupational cancers have a very long latency period—that is they do not occur until many years after exposure began; this period can be more than 30 years. Sometimes the occupational cancer is not diagnosed until after retirement, presenting a problem to investigators. This is a shortcoming of the follow-up study.

It is simply not acceptable in preventive medicine to wait and observe for years if the exposure has been present for some time. There are other ways of finding the information for an epidemiological study. One way is to collect presently available information in a case-control study, which implies knowing which disease to look for. Another alternative is the historical follow-up study.

The historical follow-up study

In this type of study the exposed and the not-exposed (the controls) are identified retrospectively. You obtain names, birth dates, social security numbers, and exposure data on people who were exposed to vinyl chloride 20 years ago and try to establish whether vinyl chloride causes cancer or not in a matter of months rather than taking years. In principle, it is not so different from the ongoing follow-up study, except that the population experience occurred in the past.

In a historical follow-up study it must be possible to match the exposure information and the disease/mortality status at an individual level. Registers of patients and deceased are therefore useful, but the information must be stored in such a way that personal identification is possible. In most countries a number of disease registers exist but there are few registers on exposures. Useful exposure information at the work site is often unfortunately thrown away.

Seek help if in doubt

Follow-up studies are expensive and time consuming as many people have to be enumerated and kept under surveillance for a long time. Usually professional help will be needed when such studies are planned and set up. The role of the work site detective will still be important in making sure that everything is going according to plan, and that all evidence is collected in a manner which will throw light on the risk of working with the exposure in question. The work site detective should also ensure that evidence is not destroyed.

Do not destroy individual exposure data

A group of exposed workers in the 1960s could form the study base together with a group of non-exposed workers, identified and followed from the 1960s until now. The number of cancer patients in the group of exposed and non-exposed could be identified via cancer registers, or in-patient registers. Alternatively you might search for cancer deaths by going through death certificates.

To summarize, a follow-up study can start when the exposure starts but also can be conducted after exposure and when disease has occurred or at some time in between. Some of the exposed can be identified before the study started, while others can enter the exposed group later on.

It is important that the non-exposed (control group) are identified at the same time as the exposed in order to make sure that both groups pass through the same observation time, it is important to have the same calendar time covered in respect of both groups.

If all workers exposed to vinyl chloride could be identified in 1960 in the plant in Kentucky, the non-exposed in the same plant in 1960 should also be identified and followed over the same period of time.

IMPORTANT CONSIDERATIONS

Dose-response

Comparing the occurrence of disease among exposed and non-exposed might be a reasonable starting point, but often the study design can be strengthened by comparing groups with different degrees of exposure. If the risk of getting the disease does increase with an increasing degree of exposure, it speaks in favour of a causal relationship between exposure and disease, Table 3.

Table 3. Relative risk of lung cancer for smokers versus non-smokers: that is, smokers' risk of getting lung cancer divided by the risk for non-smokers within a given time period

Number of cigarettes per day	Relative risk
0	1
1–4	3.7
5–15	7.5
15–24	9.6
25–49	16.6
50+	27.6

Source: Lilienfeld, A.M. (1976)

Causes and statistical association

When epidemiologists speak about risk or risk indicators, they are not necessarily speaking about causal relationship. Red haired people are at risk from skin cancer in sunny Australia, for example, not because of their red hair, but because they often lack skin protection against sunlight. The fact that people with yellow fingers run a much higher risk of lung cancer than others does not indicate that yellow fingers cause lung cancer. It is a statistical association of no causal importance. However, tobacco stained fingers are risk indicators. Risk indicators are not necessarily causes. Why do we say then that smoking is one of the causes of lung cancer as well as the cause of yellow fingers?

We say so because much of the other information we have points in that direction. For instance, we know that some of the chemical compounds in tobacco smoke produce cancer in animals. We know of a dose-response relationship—that is, heavy smokers have a higher risk of lung cancer than moderate smokers. We even have evidence which makes it unlikely that genetic factors are responsible for both the smoking habit and the risk of lung cancer.

Nevertheless, several scientists will claim that we can never know anything for sure, that there are no ways of proving a causal relationship. The scientific attitude is critical but in order to do something we do not need proofs. The detective does not have to bring about absolute proofs in court but to prove the case beyond reasonable doubt.

Even though there is a very strong association between smoking and lung cancer, the majority of even heavy smokers will not suffer from lung cancer and even a few non-smokers will acquire the disease. Therefore, tobacco smoke is not the only cause of lung cancer and tobacco smoking is not always followed by lung cancer, thus tobacco smoking is not a sufficient cause of the disease. Nevertheless, the accumulated evidence is so convincing, that most people who are familiar with the issue do think that tobacco smoke is the most frequent cause of lung cancer. In fact, we are so convinced that we have no qualms about recommending people to stop smoking.

Doing nothing also has consequences

The same rule applies in occupational medicine. Action should be taken when it is likely that the benefit of reducing exposure will do more good for the workers than the risks associated with doing nothing.

You are always having to deal with insecure premises. You act when you know enough to justify action. If you wait until you know *all* the facts you are likely to be so cautious that many workers will pay with their lives. The question is, who should benefit from the doubt, or what is the lowest level of evidence necessary to justify doing nothing.

This is well illustrated by the famous example described by John Snow (*On Cholera in London* 1855).

The most terrible outbreak of cholera which ever occurred in this kingdom, is probably that which took place in Broad Street, Golden Square, and the adjoining streets, a few weeks ago . . . As soon as I became acquainted with the situation and extent of the irruption of cholera, I suspected the water supply of the much-frequented street pump in Broad Street.

On proceeding to the spot, I found that nearly all the deaths had taken place within a short distance of the pump.

I had an interview with the Board of Guardians of St. James' parish, on the evening of Thursday, 7th September and represented the above circumstances to them. In consequence of what I said, the handle of the pump was removed on the following day.

Although the real cause of cholera was not yet known, enough was known to justify the action (and the epidemic ceased).

Objective data, subjective conclusions

Present the same set of information to a group of people and you will find they often reach different conclusions, even if they are all experts and know the subject matter well. This is even more pronounced in occupational medicine where there are conflicts of interest and money at stake. Therefore, there is no alternative than to make up your own mind and be prepared to defend your case. If the issue is important you can be sure that all the weak spots in your argument will be identified and exposed. All in occupational medicine should be familiar with at least the main problems and pitfalls in epidemiology.

PROBLEMS

It is often better to have no study than a poor study, because it is better to have an open mind than biased evidence, so do not start a study if you re not going to have confidence in the results. If you as the detective do not believe in the evidence, neither should the court.

There are many possible flaws in research and you should be familiar with some of them, much as the detective should know that burglars often leave false clues. Problems arise in many phases of research; when the study subjects are selected, when information is collected, and when data are analysed.

Selection

You plan a follow-up study and select a perfect comparison group for the exposed. Usually you will have to interview all in the study base. When the study is started you often find that not everyone wants to participate. A majority of the exposed may accept the invitation but only, say, 80 per cent of the non-exposed. If the non-respondents have a higher risk of getting the disease than the respondents, the disease frequency among the non-exposed would appear to·be lower than it was in the study base. The two groups are no longer comparable in their disease experience. We have comparability in our study base but not in our data. We have a problem of selection bias. Even a harmless exposure will seem to be associated with the disease. This evidence is worse than no evidence at all, especially if the harmless exposure might be replaced by a less 'harmless' exposure.

Information bias and misclassification

If not all of the diseased are diagnosed or if some of the diagnosed do not have the disease in the follow-up study, epidemiologists refer to information bias or misclassification. Similarly, if some of the exposed in the case-control study are classified as non-exposed, or if some of the non-exposed are registered as exposed, misclassification has occurred. If the degree of misclassification differs in the groups to be compared, the comparison could be completely meaningless.

Imagine, for instance, a case-control study, where all cases of laryngeal cancer remember a previous exposure to cutting oils, but only a proportion of the controls do. The apparent higher frequency of exposure to cutting oil among the cases will not then be real. The difference may well be due to a different threshold of recall and individuals who have developed a particular disease may be more likely to remember a possible risk factor than those who do not develop or do not have the condition.

Misclassification may occur in respect of exposure or disease, as in the previous example where cases remembered exposures better than controls. In this case the strength of the association might be overestimated, depending on the 'direction' of bias.

If misclassification of the disease state occurs independently of the exposure status in the follow-up study, the measures of association will always tend to be underestimated. An underestimated association means that the results will show values closer to 'a no association' result (RR = 1) than an 'association' result (RR ≠ 1). If the exposure classification in the case-control study is misclassified independently of the disease status, the measures of association will also be underestimated. This type of misclassification is called non-differential or random misclassification. Such types of misclassification are quite frequent and because of this many risk estimates are probably underestimated. Random misclassification is likely to occur when our industrial hygienist allocates exposures according to work histories but without knowing the disease status of the study members.

Confounding

How to select between different suspects

Most diseases have many causes. A number of occupational exposures are carcinogenic, as are tobacco smoke and other environmental pollutants. Since many of these causes produce the same disease, you cannot usually identify the relevant exposure by clinical examinations alone. The lung cancer caused by tobacco smoke looks the same as the lung cancer caused by welding fumes.

Suppose you compared the occurrence of lung cancer in those exposed to a chemical with that in a non-exposed group. You still want to make sure that what you find is not caused by, say, the different smoking habits of the groups you compared. In other words, you want to know whether smoking could be a full or partial alternative explanation for the association you may find between exposure and disease.

If, for example, the study results show a mixture of the effect of the exposure you study and tobacco smoking, epidemiologists talk about the result as being confounded. If 70 per cent of your exposed workers smoke compared with only 40 per cent of the non-exposed, then the result of the study is likely to be confounded if lung cancer is studied. The association you find could be entirely caused by smoking, or be partly caused by smoking and partly by the exposure under study. Confounding occurs when an alternative cause of the disease under study is unequally distributed among the exposure groups to be compared.

In the Kentucky example, the question of confounding is not a question of whether the workers smoked more or not. Smoking does not seem to be a cause of this particular kind of liver cancer. As a matter of fact none of the common exposures of life in the home environment could confound in this case. Instead, specific exposures—such as vinyl chloride exposure should be looked for. The workers could however have been in contact with other rare chemicals, one of which could confound the result.

Age and sex should almost always be considered as potential confounders in most studies. A large number of diseases occur with different frequencies in different age and sex groups. As long as the alternative causes of the disease are known, confounding can be avoided in several ways.

(1) Define the study base so that the alternative causes of the disease are the same for all. This is just another way of saying that exposed and not-exposed should have a similar risk of getting the disease under study, if the exposure has no causal links with the disease. Suppose the study base consists of only non-smoking males of age 45–49 years. All the people you compare should then be of the same sex, same age, and same smoking habits (non-smokers).

(2) Match the exposed and the non-exposed. For each of the exposed you select a control of the same age, sex, and life-style habits (similar background or home environment) for the disease under study.

(3) Control confounding in the data analysis. When the occurrence of the disease is finally analysed, it is carried out within subgroups of exposed and non-exposed who have the same characteristics relevant to the disease. This technique is described as stratified analysis (*see* glossary).

Although these methods of avoiding confounding often require large-scale studies, they are useful for the work place detective to know. Some of the principles can be used even in a small preliminary study.

Effect modification

Effect modification is a useful epidemiological concept, which should not be mixed up with confounding. Effect modification is when the measure of association varies between subgroups. For example, asbestos exposure is much more dangerous for smokers than for non-smokers. Looking for effect modification is another reason for carrying out stratified analysis, that is estimating the association in subgroups of the population such as smokers and non-smokers.

Effect modification is important when studying occupational exposure. You may want to know if some exposures are more harmful combined rather than separately. For example, welding stainless steel might be more dangerous for people exposed to organic solvents than for others.

Time

Diseases occur in time and the time aspect must always be kept in mind during a study. A given exposure can only 'cause' a particular disease, if the exposure occurred before the disease. Therefore, the aim of the follow-up study and the case-control study is to obtain information on exposure before the onset of the disease. In the case-control study and in the follow-up study it is important to make sure that the timing of the exposure is correct and that you have taken the time from exposure to the onset of the disease into consideration.

A number of diseases do not occur immediately after the exposure. A certain duration of exposure is necessary to start the disease process and then a certain time might elapse before the disease reaches a state where it is diagnosed by the physician or recognized by the worker. Some people call this period from the onset of exposure to diagnosis the latency period.

If it takes 10 years for a given occupational exposure to produce cancer, a study of people with less than 10 years of exposure will give no information of value. If congenital malformations are studied, the exposure data at the time of the development of the fetal organs are relevant. Exposure after that period could not cause that particular malformation.

However, it may not be possible to obtain exposure data from the relevant time period. You may only have access to present exposure and disease data. In this case a cross-sectional study may be indicated.

THE CROSS-SECTIONAL STUDY

In a cross-sectional study the occurrence (prevalence) of the disease under study for the 'exposed' is compared with the same occurrence in the non-exposed. The exposure and disease status is examined for the same time period. We do not have data to establish exposure status before the onset of the disease.

In a cross-sectional study the present work situation and present symptoms or diseases are recorded. Such a study can be carried out for all the workers in the factory, a particular section, or a sample of the workers. Data may be presented in a similar way as before (p. 27), but prevalence ratios (PR) are estimated and not relative risks, Table 4.

Table 4. Estimation of prevalence ratios

Exposure present	symptoms present		
	yes	no	all
yes	a	b	n_+
no	c	d	n_-

$$PR = \frac{a/n_+}{c/n_-}$$

This simple type of study can be very useful if the disease occurs immediately after the 'exposure' as in the case of accidents, or if the disease state does not influence the further job prospects.

A slight hearing loss, for example, is not likely to influence job prospects. Cross-sectional studies relating workers' actual hearing loss to levels of noise usually give meaningful results, showing a dose-response relationship.

In a car manufacturing plant, 57 workers were exposed to isocyanate on a certain production line. On the same production line there were 51 other non-exposed workers of similar age and sex. The study showed that two of the exposed workers had chronic bronchitis (3.5 per cent) and two among the non-exposed controls (3.9 per cent). Isocyanate did not appear to be associated with the prevalence of chronic bronchitis.

However, when the previous workers on that production line were included, there was a different result. Seven per cent of the present and past exposed workers were suffering from chronic bronchitis compared with a prevalence of 4 per cent among the non-exposed.

A cross-sectional study may help when the proportion of people on the sick list is contributed to by different departments at the factory, or if people with low back pain are classified according to their work. But caution is necessary here. Information of this kind may well be useful, but it may also be misleading. For example, you could find that bricklayers doing repair work have the highest frequency of back pain compared with other bricklayers. The reason for this is not because repair work is worse than other types of work in the trade, but simply because bricklayers with back problems tend to seek repair work which is easier to do.

Many published studies in occupational health are of the cross-sectional type. These studies can be very useful if they are carried out by those aware of their limitations; if not they can be misleading. Why then do these studies? The main place for them is when data on the timing of the exposure and the exact onset of exposure are not available. Or it might not be possible to trace people who left the factory in a given period of time. Register-based studies are often cross-sectional, as are also a number of questionnaire studies. Be sceptical when you read these papers. Many occupational diseases cannot be studied using this technique.

For example, if you want to study hand eczema among cleaners, you will almost certainly find that the longer the people have been cleaners, the fewer have hand eczema. This is simply because it is very difficult to work as a cleaner if you have skin problems, and the people who stay as cleaners for several years are likely to have a skin which can stand almost any amount of exposure to cleaning agents. (This is one aspect of the 'healthy worker' effect.)

In a cross-sectional study the occurrence of disease or ill-health is measured as a proportion of the diseased in a specific group at that specific time, a prevalence measure. This figure depends upon the number of new cases (the incidence) and the duration of the disease. The prevalence of a given disease may be high because the incidence is high or because the duration of the disease state is long—or both. An exposure which increases the incidence or prolongs the disease state will increase the prevalence. In a study using prevalence as the disease measure, you cannot usually separate risk factors from prognostic factors of disease. The prevalence of diabetes, for example, has increased in a number of countries over the past 10–20 years. This is likely to be the result of better treatment leading to long life-expectancy for diabetics rather than increasing incidence rates.

MORTALITY STUDIES

The aim of preventive medicine is to stop the cause of illness as soon as possible. So, if the study group itself is to benefit from the results, the disease state should be in an early phase.

Many published reports in occupational medicine concern mortality studies. In a follow-up study, the mortality due to a specific disease can be studied. If mortality rates among the exposed are compared with (divided by) the mortality rate for non-exposed, relative mortality rates are calculated (instead of relative morbidity rates). Often you find the term SMR (standardized mortality ratio) used in these studies, meaning that the rates are adjusted (standardized) for age-differences in the two groups compared. The SMR value gives the excess mortality in percentages. An SMR value of 130 means an excess mortality rate among the exposed of 30 per cent.

Another type of study you will often find in the literature— because of its convenience rather than quality—is the proportional mortality study (PMR).

The proportional mortality study

A number of occupational diseases lead to discomfort and lack of well-being but not to death. Other occupational diseases are of the kind that will eventually cause premature death in some people. In these instances mortality data can be used, and in most European countries mortality data are available for research.

Using mortality as the end-point is of course possible in a regular follow-up study, but you have to identify every single member of the study base back in time or sit and wait for decades to go by. If mortality data are registered at the work site, or in a pension fund, or in union records, or a similar place, a very quick and simple study can be done, and one option is the PMR study.

In this type of study, only information from the deceased is used and you only need a conceptual identification of the study base. However, you do need to identify all the deceased from that study base, which could have been in a given occupational setting over a given time period. Having done that, you at least need information from the death certificates. You need to know the causes of death and information provided by relatives or others may not be very reliable. You then calculate percentages: how many of all the deceased died of cancer? How many died of coronary heart disease? etc. Then, you compare these percentages with what you can glean from national statistical records after adjustment for age and calender period (*see* glossary).

The idea is that if a given exposure causes cancer, for example, then more people would die of cancer among the exposed compared with the non-exposed.

The proportion of cancer deaths in all those who died in the Kentucky example was higher for the vinyl chloride workers compared with the proportion of cancer deaths among all other males. If 40 per cent of all deceased exposed workers died of cancer, compared with 30 per cent among all other males, the argument is in favour of the idea that the exposure caused the cancer.

There are several problems in a study of the PMR type. The main one is that a high proportion of disease-specific mortality may appear either when the exposure is causally related to the disease, or if the exposure prevents other causes of death.

If the job prevents coronary heart disease, the proportion of cancer deaths could increase for that reason alone. If you could prevent all coronary heart disease probably 50 per cent or more of all deaths would be cancer deaths compared with the 25 per cent we see now. As a detective you would like to know if you have caught a criminal or a benefactor.

Active pilots are likely to have a low mortality from coronary heart disease since pilots at high risk of this disease (pilots with hypertension for example) are likely to be moved to other jobs or to be retired prematurely. The proportion of cancer deaths among active pilots is therefore likely to be high, even if they have a normal risk of having cancer. That is why the PMR study with an interesting result often only initiates a case-control study or a follow-up study.

It is worth mentioning that a PMR study need not be a mortality study. The same principle may be used if you have access to a disability pension register. The PMR study would then be a proportional morbidity study. Table 5 shows an example of a PMR study in a sheep-dip factory indicating a high cancer risk for the chemical workers.

Table 5. Proportion of cancer deaths of males by occupation in sheep-dip factory

Category of employment	Total deaths	Cancer deaths	Percentage of deaths due to cancer
chemical workers	41	16	39
printers, watchmen, boxmakers, carters	124	31	25

Modified from: Schilling, R.S.F. (ed). (1981).

MONITORING AND RECORD KEEPING

Epidemiology has an important role to play in occupational medicine, but there are limitations to epidemiological studies. In studying the effect of occupational exposure on the health of the workers you look at those events which you would want to have prevented.

On the other hand, not all effects on health can be foreseen and no matter how cautious you are, some exposures or some combination of exposures will turn out to be dangerous for the health of workers. When that happens, they should be detected as soon as possible in order to reduce the damage to a minimum. Epidemiology has a role to play in this process.

It is unsatisfactory that occupational causes of diseases are often recognized in a haphazard way. Too many dangerous chemicals had been around for too many years before anyone studied what happened to the exposed. This is where the idea of monitoring comes in.

In monitoring, a running system of recording health data (preferably very early signs of health effects) as well as exposure data is set up. By computing the occurrence of disease according to exposure status one hopes to be able to identify at the earliest opportunity if a given set of exposures has an influence on workers' health.

Monitoring can comprise the collection of several different types of data. Data may range from sick leave or early biological markers to death from cancer or on the exposure side, from the name of the department to the level of lead in blood.

The purpose of the monitoring system is to evaluate whether the meaures taken to protect the health of the workers are sufficient. Therefore monitoring implies a clear objective and the steps to achieve it. The monitoring process may include:

(1) Definition of the problem.
(2) Continuous data collection.
(3) Periodic analysis and interpretation.
(4) Recommendations for action.
(5) Evaluation of the action taken.

Monitoring has to be distinguished from the record keeping of data which serves a different purpose. (For example salary calculation.) It is important not to destroy any data which might give individual information on exposure, but the mere keeping of data does not mean that a proper monitoring system has been established.

Do not set up a monitoring system unless you have the personnel, skill, equipment, and time to go through all the steps in the monitoring process. Data are frequently collected and then not properly analysed. Data are sometimes analysed and no action taken. An action can be taken, but its impact never evaluated. Unused routine data from monitoring systems are by definition data of low quality. Data of low quality are of little use. Thus it is important at the beginning of the study to set up goals in monitoring, anticipate preventive strategies, and take action if the results identify a problem.

PART II

Epidemiology in practice

Examples of epidemiological 'thinking and acting' in the field of occupational health

Some of the principles of epidemiological thought have been introduced in Part I. They are mostly simple, common sense ideas. Of course there is much more to be said about each subject and some techniques will be described in more detail in the glossary. But common sense is the backbone of any study, and these examples illustrate studies which can and often should be conducted by those responsible for workers' health at the local level.

AN 'OCCUPATIONAL 'FLU' EPIDEMIC

April 15 1965; a phone call from a more than desperate manager to a department of occupational health was the beginning of the end of a puzzling situation that nearly spelled disaster for the relatively small factory that was the scene of this 'drama'.

Twenty years ago, just after the Second World War, the father of the present manager, together with two of his brothers, set up a small plant where various kinds of metal cans were manufactured. Through hard work this family business prospered and developed into a small factory, with half a dozen or so unskilled workers.

However, the demand for metal cans diminished, and it was thought worthwhile to change to a new technology. A second workshop was opened in which 'plastic' boxes were produced. The 'plastic' base material was delivered in large sheets to be cut and moulded. The manager himself and three new unskilled workers spent a week learning the technical procedures in a large factory in Germany, and production started at the end of February 1965. Initially everything went smoothly and the productivity of the workmen was considered quite good. Then things went wrong.

A fierce nationwide epidemic of influenza put practically all the workers in the metal plant as well as the new plastic workshop off work at the beginning of March. Production almost came to a standstill in the plastic section as all three of the workers and the manager had to stay at home for nearly two weeks. The three workers finally returned in the middle of March.

But then, further difficulties arose. All three workers in the plastic plant became ill once again. Their physicians' diagnosis was 'a new attack of 'flu'. Back at work, within a week they had the same symptoms of fever, headache, muscular pain, cough, wheezing; once again the sickness certificate mentioned influenza.

The manager himself, although working in close contact at the same work place, had no relapse, nor had any other worker at the metal plant. And so it went on, even in April, when no single case of 'flu occurred throughout the whole region. At this point the manager asked for advice and help.

He already had some valuable information on the situation, and he listed the notification of sickness and absence in the two sections of the factory, Table 6.

Other relevant points were as follows:

(1)   The regional influenza epidemic began at the end of February and lasted until mid-March.

Table 6. Notification of sickness—absence March to April 1965

	Worker	Number of days sickness	Number of spells	Remarks
Metal	A	8	1	
Plant	B	6	1	
	C	10	1	All absences from 1
	D	7	1	to 15 March.
	E	5	1	
	F	8	1	
Plastic	G	8/4/4	3	First spell is first
Workshop	H	7/5/3/4	4	week of March.
	I	9/4/3/5	4	Next ones in
	Manager	6	1	March/April.

(2) The sickness absence in the metal plant occurred from 1–15 March; in the plastic workshop absence went on into April.

(3) The manager himself had no symptoms of any illness after his attack of 'flu in the first week of March.

So, before starting the 'field-study' at the workshop itself, some exact data on who, when, and where were available in this case. The remaining important questions were what happened and why?

It was clear that there was something really different between the situation in the metal plant and the plastic workshop. Were those secondary and tertiary ''flu'-spells in the plastic workshop really 'flu infections? The epidemic in the region was already burnt-out. Why was the manager not affected by the ''flu' virus? What was so different between the men in the two work situations? What distinguished the three workers from the manager/co-worker? To find out, the work situation at the plastic workshop itself had to be examined more closely.

A visit to the plant was arranged without notifying the manager. The epidemiologist and the occupational toxicologist of the department of occupational health arrived at the plant on a Monday morning. The manager was very enthusiastic but extremely anxious about the possible consequences of the enquiry. In his office—a small separate room (with a non-smoking notice)—he displayed a summary of the notified sickness absence. Inquiry about the basic plastic used in the manufacture of the boxes, as indicated on the delivery documents, revealed that it was a polymer called Teflon, a polyfluorine product. The plant was typical of numerous other small workshops. On the one hand there was a very familiar lively spirit without any strict hierarchy; on the other hand a group of 10 closely-acquainted hard-working people—including the manager—were at work in a gloomy environment. Natural light filtered with difficulty through small, dust-blackened, side windows; the artificial light was poor.

The air quality was even worse. Fine particles of the cut and sawn plastic sheets filled the air. No protective devices were in use and no active dust suppression was provided at the work site itself.

The metal plant was separated from the plastic workshop because of the noise pollution emanating from the metal work. In this section the plastic dust so obvious in the other workshop was absent.

The investigators then walked around and had a chat with the workers (one of them was at home with bronchitis). They were not in a hurry and, while explaining how they carried out their job, they could smoke at ease.

At this point of the visit, the occupational toxicologist said, 'the "'flu-problem" is solved, let's have a meeting with all the workers'.

The six workers in the metal plant, two of the three occupied in the plastic workshop, and the manager met with the epidemiologist and the occupational toxicologist who took the chair.

The notification list of absences and the specific remarks, as included in the original letter referred from the manager, was the starting point for the discussion. The toxicologist explained that the Teflon sheets as such were completely harmless and inert although their constituents—monomers and other added blending compounds—could be harmful. The work procedure, as observed in the workshop, however, produced fine particles and dust. When heated, these particles would de-polymerize and release the monomers. It is these monomers which produce symptoms very similar to those of influenza.

One of the workmen pointed out that the procedure followed did not involve heating the Teflon. The chairman explained that the workers were in fact heating it with their self-rolled cigarettes. The temperature in burning cigarettes can easily reach 500°C.

That explains why the so called "'flu' relapses occurred only in the plastic plant workers and not in workers in the metal plant and why the manager, being a non-smoker, had no symptoms. The meeting ended with a decision to improve the general working conditions, to install an air exhaust system, and to make the actual work location a non-smoking area.

Remarks

1. This example illustrates how basic epidemiological principles were used on a very small sample of people. The first "'flu' epidemic caused no alarm. Everyone had 'flu so nothing pointed towards a work-related problem. Only when the "'flu' recurred several times was it obvious that a problem existed.

2. Common symptoms can mask new occupational diseases, making it difficult for physicians to identify underlying causes, when they try to use and link the information coming from the work site.

3. Using a case-control approach on just three cases and one control pointed toward tobacco smoking as a factor which occurred more frequently among diseased than not diseased. This factor could interact with the polymer fumes. That information combined with toxicological insight and literature reading solved the problem. Action was taken and the "flu" epidemic disappeared.

4. In the work environment it is sometimes not a single exposure but rather a combination of exposures or events that is important. Therefore, it is necessary to monitor or be aware of clustering of diseases, even when chemicals have been properly tested before being taken into commercial use.

5. For readers who would like to know more about this new occupational disease, we refer to Wegman and Peters (1974), and to the references in that article.

CASE STUDY OF INFERTILITY IN MALES

Setting

In 1977 a chemical factory manufactured fertilizers and pesticides for agricultural and household use. In the latter process, workers mixed, diluted, and repacked technical-grade pesticides obtained from chemical manufacturers. Some 100 different chemicals were used in the formulation of approximately 200 different products, including organophosphorus compounds, halogenated hydrocarbons and carbamates. Since 1962 the company had established a special Agricultural Chemical Division with 39 employees: three supervisors, 24 production workers, four maintenance mechanics, two clerks, and six laboratory workers. Thirty-six of the group were men.

Problem

In the 1970s the men had become increasingly aware that few of them had recently fathered children. They tried to pinpoint any differences in chemical exposure, but found that impossible since they were assigned interchangeably to different work tasks. Only the length of time they had spent in the Agricultural Chemical Division seemed to be a useful measure of exposure. They realized that seven men with long term exposure to 1,2-dibromo-3-chloropropane (DBCP) had had no children.

In the factory, DBCP was manufactured in large quantities. By informally contacting some individuals at a local university they found out that DBCP had been shown to be a mutagenic and carcinogenic agent in some experimental studies, and that there were data on reproductive effects in animals as well. Five men decided to have a sperm analysis. All of them had a low quantity of sperm (oligospermia) or no living sperm (azoospermia).

Study

At this point the workers requested a further evaluation of all employees in the group. Each of the 36 male employees was asked to complete a medical history questionaire. Semen specimens were collected from the 25 non-vasectomized males and were taken to the laboratory for determination of sperm count, motility, and morphology.

Results

Of the 25 men, 14 had azoospermia or oligospermia. Eleven men had sperm counts of less than or equal to one million/ml; 11 men had normal counts of greater than 40 million/ml; (three men had counts between 10 and 30 million/ml). The men with abnormal sperm counts had a mean exposure time of eight years: for men with normal counts the mean exposure time was 0.1 years. No worker with a sperm count of equal to or less than one million had been exposed less than three years, whereas all with a count above 40 million had been exposed less than three months.

In the factory, the airborne concentration of DBCP measured with personal air-sampling devices in early 1977 was 0.4 ppm (average over an eight-hour day).

Impact of study

The results described led to a lowering of the threshold limit value (TLV) and to the instigation of further studies. It also started a debate within the scientific community, the regulatory agencies, and the public at large.

New studies

A second study at the same factory was conducted in which an attempt was made to study testicular function in all male employees. The total male population at risk was 310. Of these only 142 provided semen samples, 107 were classified as 'ever' exposed and 35 were classified as 'never' exposed. For the 'ever' exposed group the median sperm count was 46 million/ml: for the 'never' exposed group the median count was 79 million/ml. Of the exposed workers 13 per cent were azoospermic, 17 per cent were severely oligospermic, and 16 per cent mildly oligospermic. Among the non-exposed workers, 3 per cent were azoospermic, none severely oligospermic, and 6 per cent mildly oligospermic.

As a result of these findings, several other studies were conducted of workers at other DBCP manufacturing facilities. Agricultural workers who used the chemicals were also studied. These studies were important because they showed DBCP effects on spermatogenesis at levels of exposure potentially lower than those observed in the production process.

The debate

The chemical suspected to be the cause of infertility had in 1961 been shown to be toxic in the tests on rats, guinea pigs, and rabbits. Furthermore, carcinogenicity and mutagenicity of DBCP in animals had been established in 1973 and 1975. Nevertheless the problem of infertility in humans was first identified by a group of concerned workers. So, even if the effects of DBCP were known to the scientific community, the workers and the people responsible for their health were not informed of them.

Long-term effect

After substitution of DBCP, workers who were azoospermic did not regain the ability to produce sperm. However, the sperm counts of most of those who were oligospermic did improve considerably.

Remarks

1. This example clearly underlines the importance of workers' experience. It also shows that new diseases may arise when new chemicals are introduced on the market.

2. New chemicals should be tested in short-term tests and in animal studies before workers are exposed; but it is of little help if the test results are not used or known by the workers or the people in charge of their health.

3. Most of the studies mentioned in the example were carried out by professional researchers, but those locally involved could have come far by using simple methods. By defining the problems the workers had discussed among themselves, fertility could have been identified as the issue to be examined. A short questionnaire study would, for example, have shown that the workers exposed to DBCP had fewer children than the rest of the workers and that more of them were involuntarily childless.

   (Simple ways of calculating expected fertility were even worked out as a result of this study: Levine R.J. *et al.* (1980).)

   It would also have been possible at the local level to get sperm counts from the 25 DBCP workers and recognize the dose-response pattern by plotting sperm counts versus exposure duration.

4. All personal data (including those on fertility) must be considered confidential. Nevertheless, if the workers had not been willing to share their experience with others, then the cause of the infertility could not have been identified and disease prevention would not have been possible.

5. A case-control study was the first approach (as it often is) in identifying the cause of the disease. Results were later confirmed in follow-up studies where fertility among other

exposed workers was compared with unexposed. The cohort of exposed workers was identified as far back in time as possible according to available records. Such studies are often referred to as historical or retrospective follow-up studies.

6. Non-respondents are frequent in many epidemiological studies including the present one where only 142 out of 310 workers provided semen samples. Non-response will often introduce bias (a systematic error) in the results of the study, but the magnitude of the bias will depend upon the reasons for which people refuse to participate. If these reasons are unrelated to both the exposure and the disease status no bias will occur. In this study the effect of DBCP exposure on sperm production was so obvious that bias is hardly the only explanation.

7. There are several causes of low sperm count which were considered in the study. None of these differed between the diseased and the not diseased.

A SMALL CLUSTER OF SPONTANEOUS ABORTIONS

At a small factory close to a town in a rural area, about 40 women were mainly engaged in sewing men's shirts. The work was monotonous and badly paid. Previously, most women only stayed in the job for a short period of time and left when other work opportunities presented. However, because of a high rate of unemployment among unskilled women in the area, these 40 women had been at the factory from two to ten years. They knew each other well, not only because they worked together, but also because most of them lived within a short distance of the factory in a sparsely populated area. Thirty-two of the women were under 45 years of age. One day the factory nurse was contacted personally by one of the women. She told her that she and her husband had been trying to have a child for some time. When she had finally become pregnant, she had lost the child after about three months. She had discussed the matter with some of the other women at the work place, and three others reported that they had also had a spontaneous abortion within the last two years.

Was there an excess of spontaneous abortion?

First, the nurse checked to see if the observed number of spontaneous abortions exceeded the expected number. This preliminary expected number was calculated on the assumption that the women in question had the same risk of spontaneous abortions as all other women.

The nurse tried to verify that she had identified all abortions and that the abortions were in fact spontaneous and not induced. She asked if the abortions were diagnosed by a physician, or if they had led to hospitalization. Then she identified the study base which in this case is the number of women in the work area who had been pregnant in the last two years. That is, all women who gave birth to a child, and those who had had an abortion, spontaneous or provoked.

Whilst making this inquiry, the factory nurse found that, in the past two years, 12 of the women currently employed had been pregnant. Four had had a spontaneous abortion, and three had been hospitalized for that reason. The remaining eight had given birth to a child. None reported any induced abortions during the last two years. This meant that 33 per cent of the recognized pregnancies ended as spontaneous abortions and 25 per cent ended as hospitalized spontaneous abortions. It was then necessary to compare these percentages with the expected figure for the community at large.

By checking statistical reports the nurse saw that an overall rate of hospitalized spontaneous abortions of 10 per cent was expected. By reading some of the literature in the field, she learned that the proportion of spontaneous abortions, based upon self-reported cases came to 12–14 per cent, much less than the observed number.

No specific data were available for the special geographical region of the work site and no data existed for the social class in question. The pregnant women had an age distribution similar to that of pregnant women in the country at large, so there was no need to adjust the expected number.

Was the factory nurse faced with a work-related problem?

Assessing the information, the nurse concluded that the observed number of spontaneous abortions exceeded the expected number, but this might have been due to many non occupational factors, such as: selection or confounding—that is, caused by other exposure or intrinsic factors, or chance. She had to rule out as many of these other explanations as possible. If none of these explanations was likely, she could have been facing a work-related problem.

Selection

At this preliminary stage, the women at this particular work site were compared with women of the same age in the same country. This is a crude comparison and the two groups may not be comparable for several reasons. For instance, if pregnant women leave work late in pregnancy, this would of course overestimate the abortion rate among workers, if such women were not included in the study. The numerator would be the same since spontaneous abortions occur early in pregnancy, but the denominator would be less than it should be. The group of machinists and the women of the whole country would not therefore be comparable. However, no such explanation was found to operate in this case.

More subtle forces of selection are likely to distort the comparability of the two groups. Women with small children at home would be less likely to have work outside the home. These women might be in a low risk group, since they had recently demonstrated their reproductive capability. Controlling factors of this sort is beyond the scope of a study at the work site level. This should be left to the professional epidemiologists. Before the nurse handed over the investigation to the researchers, there were several other things to be done. Some information on the aetiology of spontaneous abortion was required from the medical library.

Confounding: looking for alternative explanations

The nurse found out that surprisingly little was known about the aetiology of spontaneous abortion. Most of the early spontaneous abortions have chromosomal abnormalities; therefore exposures which could damage the genetic structures—either directly in the fetus or indirectly through the germ-cells of the father or mother— could lead to spontaneous abortions. Which exposures, other than the ones at the work site, or what alternative explanation could explain the excess of spontaneous abortions?

Did the women have any exposure in common which should be taken into consideration? Did they share the same water supply? Did they live close to each other and if so, was there any risk of, for example, air pollution in the area? Had they had any similar contagious disease early in pregnancy? Had they received any medical treatment? Were they all heavy smokers? Did they consume large quantities of alcohol? What occupations did their husband have? etc.

In this case none of the four women, who had the spontaneous abortions, had had any of the above exposures in common. Two of the women were pregnant for the first time. For all the women it was their first spontaneous abortion. None had any serious diseases, neither did their husbands have any particular exposures in common. The nurse therefore had to conclude that there was no obvious explnation.

Having considered alternative explanations, the nurse focused on possible causes at the work site.

Studies at the work site

It was simple to note that all four women involved were working in the sewing machine department, distributed throughout the work area. However, most of the other women who had been pregnant also worked in the same room. Three of the four women had worked on shift work during pregnancy, compared with 40 per cent of the other women who had a child during the study period. All had been engaged in welding of a PVC raincoat material. Only two of the other pregnant women had been in the same work process. None had been pregnant within the last two years. Production of raincoats only began a year and a half ago.

None of those in the area were exposed to organic solvents, heavy metals, or any other harmful substance. No other chemical substance could leak from any other area of the factory to the sewing area through the ventilation system.

Chance

Even if the women working at the particular work site in the long run had a risk of spontaneous abortion close to the average, the rate would sometimes be above average, sometimes less than average. The number of spontaneous abortions is not a fixed proportion of all pregnancies. It fluctuates, as do most biological phenomena, for unknown reasons which we often call 'chance'.

If the nurse had access to data from previous time periods, and if these data showed a high number of spontaneous abortions compared with the expected number, it would suggest an association not rooted in chance. However, a previously normal rate is of course no proof that the clustering of spontaneous abortions is the result of chance.

It would indicate rather that the nurse should be aware of any changes in the work process, which had taken place within recent years.

The chance possibility is one which always remains when other possibilities have been ruled out. Obviously the larger the study the less likely it is that chance will distort the results to a large extent.

Conclusion

The nurse had now used a number of epidemiological techniques, and had practised a good deal of epidemiological thinking; she had not proved anything. The four spontaneous abortions could easily have been a chance phenomenon. Nevertheless she had identified a situation where an excess of spontaneous abortions, whether due to chance or not, had occurred. The production of plastic raincoats needed to be checked carefully. A larger study should be designed and she should be able to convince an epidemiologist that such a study was worth while and necessary.

The professional epidemiologist would probably not only expand the study base to other women with similar exposure, but also expand the outcomes to be measured. If possible infertility, spontaneous abortions, low birthweight, premature births, and congenital malformations should be included in further studies.

Remarks

1. Quite often no immediate solution will be found because a clustering of disease could be a purely chance phenomenon. But the proper attitude is to assume that the problem is real

until substantial evidence indicates the opposite. The exposed should be given 'the benefit of the doubt'.

2. Again simple epidemiological principles were used to quantify the potential problem. The case-control approach helped to identify possible exposures of interest, by comparing working conditions and other habits and exposures between the women who had spontaneous abortions (cases) and women with normal pregnancies (controls).

3. The number of women in this study is far too small to 'prove' anything, but it provides an important report of a cluster. A full-scale investigation is certainly called for.

4. As mentioned before, only a small number of spontaneous abortions occurred. If statistical-significance testing (a test that would state the probability of the excess finding of spontaneous abortions, had it occurred by chance alone) had been performed, no significant result would have been found (no result with such a probability less than 5 per cent). However, lack of statistical significance is no 'proof' of lack of cause-effect relationships.

5. Epidemiologists are mainly interested in groups of people rather than in individuals. Therefore the first part of any epidemiological study will usually be to compare the observed number of cases with what would have been expected in a similar non-exposed group of people. If an excess is identified, the next step is to look for its reasons. These may be due to bias, for instance or to selection, other habits or exposures which would explain the excess (confounding) or exposure at the work site.

6. The pregnant women in the work area had an age distribution similar to that of pregnant women in the country at large, so no immediate need for age adjustment seemed necessary. Usually adjustment for age or for other variables which may differ between the two groups being compared (case-controls; exposed, non-exposed) is necessary (*see* age standardization in the glossary).

BYSSINOSIS AND CHRONIC BRONCHITIS IN
A FLAX-MILL

In January 1965 a member of a trade union was delegated by his organization to ask for advice on an alleged health problem in two flax-weaving mills. As the plants had at that time no organized health service, the workers union took the initiative and made contact with the occupational health department of the nearby medical faculty.

The two weaving mills processed dry spun flax producing heavy linen canvas for tent material; they had been in operation for about 15 years. Many, but not all, of the workmen in the plant complained of an irritating cough and wheezing which they said was caused by the flax dust. The plant owners, on the other hand, complained of a disturbingly high absence rate—especially on Mondays—and a huge turnover of staff. They produced a list of 194 persons who had left the plant in the last 15 years.

The physician in the department of occupational health could easily agree with the workers' hypothesis that the flax dust was the cause of the chest complaints. It is well known that inhalation of flax dust may provoke a specific broncho-pulmonary disease, called byssinosis.

The research team organized a meeting with the workers' delegate, the engineer, the chief technician, and the head of administration. There was an agreement to study lung disease among the work force and if necessary to suggest environmental improvements at the plant.

Study

All workers at the two mills were questioned about chest complaints and out of 155 workers, 28 were diagnosed as having byssinosis. Since the administration had a list of all 194 persons who had left the plant in the last 15 years, it was also possible to study those who had left the factory. Fifty-two of them could not be traced, but of the remaining 142, 79 were diagnosed as having byssinosis.

The proportion of cases with the disease was much higher (56 per cent) among workers who had left the factory than among workers still employed at the plant (18 per cent). It was obvious that selection had taken place and that turnover had been partly determined by having developed the disease.

Remarks

1. In this example the aetiology of the symptoms was clear from the beginning. The purpose of the study was not to elaborate causal hypotheses but rather to estimate the size of the problem. Another task was to monitor the health and safety record at the plant which turned out to be unsatisfactory.

2. In a situation like this it is obvious that improvements in the working conditions should be initiated immediately. The study should not be made an excuse to delay necessary action.

3. The study is of the cross-sectional type and it is the prevalence of byssinosis which is studied. The limitations of cross-sectional studies would have been even more apparent had the study base been restricted to present workers, as is often the case.

CASE STUDY IN A POWER PLANT

In March 1979 the factory inspectorate received a letter from a group of unions who had received by mail a number of reports from several power plants. These reports gave details of premature deaths from cardiovascular disease among union workers.

In two plants, employing about 250 union members, there had been 20 deaths in a 12 year period. The average age of the deceased was 60 years and the average length of employment was 14–16 years. In another plant there had been 28 deaths in the period 1968–78 and 70 per cent of the deceased were union members. Union members, however, only accounted for one-third of the total employed at the power plant.

In the letter it was stressed that the workers were often exposed to noise and vibration, and the union asked for a further investigation of the problem. It was obvious that the data presented in the letter were interesting, but much information was lacking. Had the cause of deaths been a very rare disease, the data might have been sufficient to convince the reader that a work-related problem did exist. However, cardiovascular diseases are not rare causes of death. On the contrary, this group of diseases constitutes the most common cause of death amongst adult men.

Study

The expected number of deaths from cardiovascular disease in a population of a similar age structure to the employed power plant workers should be available from national statistics. It would then be necessary to identify all the deaths of plant workers and their causes and to extract those due to cardiovascular disease. The number of deaths due to cardiovascular disease is then divided by the total number of deaths amongst power plant workers and compared with the expected rate (*see* glossary).

Results

The observed proportion of cardiovascular deaths was actually less than the proportion found among all deceased males in the country that is, the observed was similar to the expected.

Discussion

There are at least three possible and related explanations for this.

(1) The results would be expected if no occupational risks of cardiovascular disease operated at the power plants.

(2) Working at the power plant increased the risk of cardiovascular and other diseases. In spite of an increased mortality rate, the proportion of all deaths will remain unchanged.

(3) A badly selected comparison group was used—this is an example of healthy worker selection. Full-time employment implies good health, and people with severe chronic diseases are not likely to work at a power plant.

Further study on this would probably be beyond the scope of a work-site investigation. Investigations by professional epidemiologists should try to exclude explanations 2 and 3.

New studies

A proportional mortality study was conducted, using data from basic vital statistics as a reference. A more satisfactory comparison group of other employed workers was selected, and there were still no excess deaths from cardiovascular disease. The third explanation then seemed unlikely.

All employed workers at a number of power plants were then identified in a given time period. The observed mortality in the group was tallied, and the expected mortality was calculated using mortality rates from the general population and other employed groups. Again no excess risk of cardiovascular disease was found and the second explanation did not seem to be likely. Further studies were not planned.

Conclusion

No extra risk for cardiovascular disease in power plants could be detected.

Remarks

1. Record-keeping is very important in epidemiological studies. If the necessary data are available for research, important questions may be answered in a short time span.
2. By using already existing data, little work was needed to work out a proportional mortality ratio. In spite of the limitations of PMR studies, the insights obtained were later confirmed by a more appropriate study.
3. In this example, the reference group is used to estimate the expected cardiovascular mortality among the power plant workers. If no occupational hazards existed a mortality ratio of 1 should be expected. Quite often values less than 1 are found, due to lack of comparability between workers and the general population. This is the healthy worker effect mentioned in the example.

LUNG CANCER MORTALITY AMONG WORKERS
EXPOSED TO CHROMATE PIGMENTS

Motivation for study

Workers involved in the manufacture of zinc and lead chromate pigments drew the attention of the occupational physician to several fatal cases of lung cancer among their co-workers. The occupational physician in charge of this small plant (92 workers) first noted that all the cases were smokers and considered that the condition was not related to occupation.

In 1974 two new cases and in 1976 a third one changed that point of view and the physician decided to consult the Institute of Occupational Medicine to set up a study to determine if an occupational hazard was involved.

Study and results

All 251 workers who had worked for six months or more in the plant between 1958 and 1978 were included in the study. Occurrence and dates of death were obtained from the plant or death registers or both. Causes of death could not be obtained from death certificates in the country where the study was conducted and were therefore obtained from families, physicians, hospitals, or pathologists.

Lung cancer mortality was compared with local lung cancer mortality among men, using numbers of deaths obtained from the National Institute of Medical and Health Research and demographic data from the 1954, 1962, 1968, and 1975 censuses. In all cases 10 year age bands were used.

Of the total of 53 deaths among workers at the plant, only 32 causes could be ascertained, and 13 of these were cases of lung cancer. Assuming that none of the unknown causes of death was due to lung cancer, this number was compared with the expected number of 2.6, which is based on the lung cancer mortality rate in the general population. The five fold excess of observed to expected was large and statistically significant.

Had the basic risk of lung cancer deaths amongst the workers in fact been similar to what was seen for others of similar age and sex, the probability of this excess being due to random fluctuations alone was small, less than five per cent.

After the study

Chrome exposure in this plant had always exceeded the allowed maximum level, the threshold limit value of 50 mg/m^3. It was considered from the results of the follow-up study and comparable studies in other countries leading to similar results that this exposure was responsible for the excess number of cases of lung cancer. This was recognized officially and cases of lung cancer after exposure to zinc and lead chromate pigments were therefore accepted for compensation according to the regulations.

Workers at the plant were informed of the results of the survey. Exposure levels in the environment as well as in the blood and urine of workers were determined. They showed that environmental levels were occasionally extremely high (more than 2000 mg/m^3). Blood and urine levels were also high. High risk posts were automated; or exposure was reduced to less than 50 mg/m^3 using ventilation equipment. Nine workers used masks.

It was decided to monitor the death rate from lung cancer in this plant to check whether the protective measures were relevant and efficient in eliminating the risk of lung cancer in the plant.

Remarks

1. Fortunately, all records on employees were kept and could be used in a historical follow-up study.

2. However, only a fraction (32/53) of the causes of death could be identified, but the study still provided useful information.

3. It is likely that some of the unknown causes of death were due to lung cancer. If so the true ratio of observed to expected would have been even higher and the SMR presented by the investigators would have been an underestimate.

4. The occupational physician in charge of the plant first noted that all cases were smokers and considered that the health problems were not related to occupation. Keep in mind that in spite of the fact that smoking is an important cause of lung cancer, still the majority of smokers will never develop lung

cancer. Smoking is not the only cause of lung cancer. Disregarding the role of occupational factors because of workers' smoking habits is common, but often unreasonable. To be a confounder smoking must be more frequent among the exposed compared to the non-exposed, and even if they did confound, smoking habits have to be very different to explain a large excess of risk (Axelson 1978).

5. Smoking may interact with occupational exposures (such as asbestos) to increase the damage caused.

6. The evaluation of protective measures should always be part of an epidemiological investigation, particularly in this example, where the carcinogen is still in the work environment.

Glossary

Aetiological fraction (*see* Attributable risk)

Aetiology (causality)

The mechanism which relates causes to the diseases (or symptoms) they produce.

Attributable proportion (*see* Attributable risk)

Attributable risk

The fraction of disease attributable to an exposure within a population. Such a population may be the exposed one (attributable risk among the exposed) or the general population (attributable risk in the population). It is the proportion of the disease that would be eliminated should the incidence in the exposed group be reduced to the level of the unexposed group.

The most simple formulas for attributable risks in the population (AR_p) and among exposed (AR_c) are:

$$AR_p = \frac{\text{Proportion of exposed } (RR - 1)}{\text{Proportion of exposed } (RR - 1) + 1}$$

$$AR_c = \frac{RR - 1}{RR}$$

RR = Relative risk, relative rate

Example: If people exposed to organic solvents have an incidence rate of chronic brain damage three times that of those not exposed, and if 1 per cent of the population is exposed, the attributable risk (AR_p) will be:

$$AR_p = \frac{0.01 \times (3 - 1)}{0.01 \times (3 - 1) + 1} = 0.02$$

In this example, 2 per cent of chronic brain damage can be prevented in the population if solvent exposure is eliminated.

Among the exposed only, the attributable risk will be

$$AR_c = \frac{3-1}{3} = 0.67.$$

Thus 67 per cent of chronic brain damage in this group could be prevented by eliminating the exposure.

Bias

A systematic error which can occur during the design, conduct, and interpretation of an investigation. Bias will cause results to depart from true values. There are several types of bias.

An example could be recall bias. Mothers of children with a congenital malformation may be more likely than mothers of healthy newborns to remember details of chemical exposures during pregnancy. A higher frequency of exposures to chemicals in the mothers of malformed children would then be expected. That is, an association between fetal exposure to chemicals and malformations would exist in our data, even if in reality the two groups had been equally exposed.

Case-control study

The study in which the distribution of exposure amongst diseased (e.g. incident cases) is compared with the exposure distribution amongst a proper reference group (amongst people without the disease at the time of case selection).

The simplest possible presentation of the results of such a case-control study is:

Exposure	Cases	Controls
+	a	b
−	c	d
Total	n_+	n_-

The estimate of the incidence rate among exposed, divided by the incidence rate amongst non-exposed (RR), is given by the odds ratio (OR):

$$OR = \frac{a/c}{b/d} \quad \frac{ad}{cb}$$

Case-control study within a cohort

Case-control study where the study base is a cohort followed over time. The exposure status of the cohort members with the disease (the cases) is compared with the exposure status in the study base in a sample of the non-diseased (the controls).

Case-group

The group of people in the study base with the disease or health disorder under investigation.

Causes

Determinants of diseases or ill health (in epidemiology). A cause is termed necessary when it always precedes an effect. A sufficient cause always initiates or produces an effect.

Cluster

A number of persons or things gathered or situated close together. A *disease cluster* is then a number of diseased gathered close together in place, such as in a factory, or in time. In epidemiology a cluster of diseases usually refer to an excess of cases, or a high incidence of cases in a given population.

Cohort

A group of people with one or more features in common, e.g. year of birth, type of exposure, employment in a given factory over a given period of time. In more general terms, any of such groups of people followed over a period of time.

Cohort study (*see* Follow-up study)

Confounder

An alternative cause, or a correlate of it, of the disease under study which is more frequent (or less frequent) among exposed compared with the non-exposed. Leads to confounding if not properly dealt with in the study.

Confounding

An observed association which is partly or totally the result of an association with another factor, an alternative cause of a disease or a correlate of such another cause. The estimate of the link between exposure and disease is mixed with the link between the disease and another factor (the confounder).

Control group

A comparison group. In the follow-up study it is the group of not-exposed which is used to estimate the expected disease occurrence among the exposed, had they not been exposed. In the case-control study it is the group which is used for estimating the exposure distribution in the study base (the reference group).

Cross-sectional study

Case-control and cohort/follow-up studies have (longitudinal) recording of exposure and onset of disease in time. At least the exposure is known to have been present before the disease occurred. In the cross-sectional study disease as well as exposure is recorded at one particular point in time. The simplest possible presentation of the results of a cross-sectional study is:

Exposure	Diseased	Non-diseased	Total
+	a	b	m_+
−	c	d	m_-
Total	n_+	n_-	n

Since disease (and exposure) is only measured at one point in time only prevalence can be measured. The relative prevalence rate (PR) or the prevalence rate difference (PD) are:

$$PR = \frac{a/m_+}{c/m_-} \qquad\qquad PD = a/m_+ - c/m_-$$

Dose-response relationship

A relationship in which a change in exposure is associated with a change in the occurrence of the disease under study.

Effect modification

A factor that modifies the effect of a causal factor under study. The measure of association varies in subgroups. The measure may for example be stronger (or weaker) for males than for females, or for smokers than for non-smokers, etc. Effect modification is part of the concept of interaction.

Excess rate (*see* Rate difference)

Follow-up

Observation over time of an individual, a group, or a defined population in order to record changes in health status during the follow-up period.

Follow-up study

In the follow-up study a group of exposed and a group of not-exposed are followed over time and the occurrence of disease is measured in these two groups. The simplest possible presentation of the results of a follow-up study is:

Exposure	Diseased	Non-diseased	Persons	Total Person-time
+	a	b	m_+	t_+
−	c	d	m_-	t_-

Incidence rates and risks can be calculated directly, and the formulae for the most common-used measures of association are:

Relative rate/Rate ratio (RR) $= \dfrac{a/t_+}{c/t_-}$

Relative risk (RR) $= \dfrac{a/m_+}{c/m_-}$

Rate difference (RD) $= a/t_+ - c/t_-$

Risk difference (RD) $= a/m_+ - c/m_-$

Incidence rate

Incidence rate is the basic measure of disease frequency and is defined as:

$$\frac{\text{Number of new cases of the disease that occurs in a population at risk during a given time period}}{\text{Sum of the length of time at risk of getting the disease for each individual in the population (person time).}}$$

Suppose that among the workers of a factory, there are three cases of cancer of the stomach between 1975 and 1985. The denominator is defined as the length of time that each individual is at risk of getting the disease and is measured in person time.

Example: The factory opened in the beginning of 1975 with 100 workers. Five of those 100 workers died at the beginning of 1979 from causes other than stomach cancer. An additional 300 workers were first employed at the beginning of 1983.

The five people who died in 1979 were not at risk of developing stomach cancer after they had died and the 300 workers first employed in the factory in 1983 were only at risk of developing stomach cancer as workers in the factory after that time. The three cases of stomach cancer (diagnosed at the beginning of 1978, 1981, 1984 respectively all belonged to the first employed) were only at risk of developing the condition whilst they were free of it. For simplicity consider all events to have taken place on 1 January each year.

The sum for each individual in the population of the lengths of time at risk of getting stomach cancer will be:

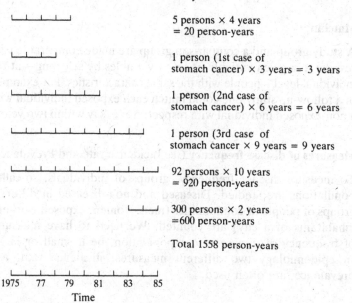

5 persons × 4 years
= 20 person-years

1 person (1st case of
stomach cancer) × 3 years = 3 years

1 person (2nd case of
stomach cancer) × 6 years = 6 years

1 person (3rd case of
stomach cancer × 9 years = 9 years

92 persons × 10 years
= 920 person-years

300 persons × 2 years
=600 person-years

Total 1558 person-years

1975   77   79   81   83   85
Time

Our incidence rate will then be 3/1558 person-years or two new cases of stomach cancer/1000 person-years.

Note: Person-years represent person-time, not persons. The sum of 100 person-years could represent 10 persons observed for 10 years each, or 20 persons observed for five years each.

Interaction

The interdependent operation of two or more causes to produce an effect (*see also* effect modification).

Latency

The time period between exposure to an agent causing a disease and the appearance of manifestations of the disease. For example in a study of bladder cancer in people exposed to aromatic amines, the time between first exposure and onset of disease was on average 18 years.

Matching

A study group and a comparison group are made comparable with respect to a given variable or set of variables by selecting—at the individual level—people with the same characteristics. For example, in a follow-up study one could match each exposed individual with a non-exposed individual with respect to age, say within two years.

Measures of disease frequency (*see* Incidence rate and Prevalence)

To measure disease frequency, groups of individuals: so-called populations are studied. Diseased and non-diseased in different groups of people or communities (men, women, exposed workers, inhabitants of a city) are counted. We need to have measures of frequency of disease in our population, be it small or large. In epidemiology two different measures, incidence rate, and prevalence, are often used.

Misclassification

The erroneous classification of an individual into a disease or exposure category other than that to which it he or she should be assigned. If the probability of misclassification varies between compared groups (differential misclassification) the biased measure of association can be an over- or an underestimation of the effect. If the probability of misclassification is the same in all study groups (non-differential or random misclassification) the measure of effect is always underestimated.

Odds ratio (OR)

The ratio of two odds (the probability of occurrence of an event to that of non occurrence). In a case-control study the OR is calculated as an exposure-odds ratio, such as:

Exposure	Disease	No disease
yes	*a*	*b*
no	*c*	*d*

$$OR = \frac{a/c}{b/d} \quad \frac{ad}{cb}$$

The odds ratio is then the ratio of the odds in favour of exposure among cases (a/c) to the odds in favour of exposure among non cases (b/d). This odds ratio estimates the relative risks under a given set of assumptions depending upon sample selection of cases and controls, or the frequency of disease.

Prevalence

Prevalence is the proportion of people who have a disease (or a characteristic) at a given point in time. To compute it, divide the number of people with the disease by the number of people in the population of interest. For instance, 50 people have chronic bronchitis in an employed population of 1000 people, then the prevalence will be:

$$p = \frac{\text{number of individuals having the disease at a given time}}{\text{number of individuals in the population at that given time}}$$

$$= \frac{50}{1000} = 0.05 \text{ or } 5\%.$$

Note that the prevalence is a *proportion* because the numerator is included in the denominator.

Proportion

A type of ratio in which the numerator is included in the denominator $A/(A + B)$. A proportion multiplied by 100 describes the number of cases with a particular characteristic expressed as a percentage of all.

Example: Out of 86 workers examined for hearing loss, 26 have a deficit in hearing and 60 did not. The proportion of people with deficit in hearing is $26/(26 + 60) = 26/86 = 0.30$ or 30%.

Proportional mortality ratio

The proportion of deaths from a specific disease in a given time period out of all deaths in the same time period.

The technique of computing an age adjusted PMR value is rather similar to computing an SMR (standardized mortality ratio). As in SMR (see page 81), the total number of observed deaths is divided by the total number expected to give a proportional mortality ratio.

To compute an age-adjusted PMR:

1. Count the number of deaths by age at deaths for all causes.

Observed deaths by age at death

	25–34	35–44	45–54	55–64	65–74	Total
All causes	3	8	18	29	51	109

2. Count the number of deaths for the disease of interest, e.g. lung cancer.

Observed death of lung cancer by age at death

	25–34	35–44	45–54	55–64	65–74	Total
Lung cancer	1	3	7	14	18	43

3. Calculate the number of expected deaths due to lung cancer as if the proportion of cancer deaths would have been the same as in the general population. By multiplying this proportion by the total number of deaths (all causes) in each group and summing up the results, the number of expected deaths is reached.

Age at death

	25–34	35–44	45–54	55–64	65–74	Total
Proportion of lung cancer death in the general population	0.180	0.218	0.270	0.302	0.270	
Expected deaths for lung cancer	3×0.180 = 0.5	8×0.218 = 1.7	8×0.270 = 4.9	29×0.302 = 8.8	51×0.270 = 13.8	29.7

The ratio of observed over expected deaths multiplied, by convention, by 100 gives us the age adjusted proportional mortality ratio:

$$PMR = \frac{43}{29.7} \times 100 = 144$$

A PMR of 100 indicates that the proportion of deaths from cancer is the same in the study group and in the general population. A PMR above 100 indicates more lung cancer deaths than expected. This PMR shows that the proportion of cancer mortality (out of all causes of death) in this group is 44 per cent above the population level. This could be due to a high lung cancer mortality or to a low, eg. cardiovascular mortality. The PMR value is a much less intelligible measure of association than the SMR value.

Rate

A measure of the number of events occurring during a particular time. In the medical literature a rate measures deaths or occurrence of diseases during some specified period. A rate is a ratio in which the number of health events is divided by observation time.

Example: if 80 new cases of lung cancer occurred in a *cohort* during 35 000 person-years of experience, the *incidence rate* of lung cancer will be 80/35 000 person-years or 229/100 000 person-years. (*See also*: *Incidence rate*, *Prevalence*.)

Sometimes one may find an incidence rate as the number of new diseased in a given population over a time period of one year divided by the number of individuals in the population. In this case the denominator is still an estimate of observation time.

Rate difference

The difference between two rates. For example, the difference in incidence rate between a population exposed to a factor and a population not exposed. The term excess rate may be used as a synonym for rate difference.

Example: in a study of mortality of lung cancer among smokers and non-smokers the incidence rate among the smokers is 104 new deaths from lung cancer every 100 000 smoking person-years. The incidence rate among the non-smokers is 10 new deaths from lung cancer every 100 000 non-smoking person-years. The rate difference is 104/100 000 − 10/100 000 = 94/100 000.

This rate is the excess rate due to smoking.

Ratio

The value obtained by dividing one quantity by another. Rates, proportions, percentages are all ratios.

Example: in a group of people we observe 109 deaths while 70 deaths were expected if our group had the mortality rates as the *Reference population*. The ratio of observed to expected deaths is 109/70 = 1.56.

Reference population

The population which is used as a comparison for the population under study.

Relative rate

The ratio of two rates. For example the incidence or mortality rate in the exposed population divided by the similar rate for the non-exposed.

Relative risk

The ratio of the risk of disease or death among the exposed to the risk among those not exposed.

Risk

A probability that an event will occur, e.g. that an individual will become ill or die within a stated period of time.

Example: a man who smokes a pack of cigarettes a day, starting at 18 years has a risk of approximately 10 per cent of dying of lung cancer before he reaches the age of 65.

Standardization

The standardized mortality ratio (SMR) is standardized according to the age distribution among the exposed. The principle of standardization can of course also be applied to other characteristics.

Example: results from a cross-sectional study could be stratified according to sex in the following way:

Sex	Exposure	Diseased	Total	Relative Prevalence Rates
M	+	20	100	
	−	5	50	2.0
F	+	5	50	
	−	5	100	2.0
Total	+	25	150	
	−	10	150	2.5

The table shows that the relative prevalence is 2.0 for males and females, but 2.5 for the total group (bottom line). The result for the total group is due to confounding. Males have a higher prevalence of the disease than females, and more males are exposed.

By applying the standardization principle we could work out the expected number of diseased among the exposed had they had the same prevalence as the non-exposed and a similar distribution of males and females.

It is seen that 10 per cent of non-exposed males have the disease (5 out of 50) and 5 per cent of females (5 out of 100). Therefore 10 per cent of 100 exposed males would be expected to have the disease, in the absence of exposure (10 males), and 5 per cent of the 50 exposed females (2.5 females). The total number of expected diseased would then add up to 12.5, which could be compared with the 25 observed cases. A sex-standardized prevalence ratio would then be $25/12.5 = 2.0$.

Standardized mortality ratio (SMR)

Population mortality rates are often used as a basis of comparison for the number of observed deaths in a specific group. A standardized mortality ratio is computed as follows:

1. The number of observed deaths in the occupational group of interest is tallied. Since mortality rates are age and sex dependent, observed mortality is usually counted by age for one sex at a time.

Observed deaths by age at death

25–34	35–44	45–54	55–64	65–74
3	8	18	29	51

2. The number of expected deaths is estimated by using age specific mortality rates for the general population. For instance, general population mortality rates per 1000 persons at risk per year, might be:

Mortality rates by age

25–34	35–44	45–54	55–64	65–74
0.933	2.013	6.810	18.774	48.852

To calculate the number of expected deaths among our workers had they had the same death rate as the population at large, person-years of observation in different age groups must be worked out.

Person-years of observation by age

25–34	35–44	45–54	55–64	65–74
1600y	2000y	1700y	1000y	700y

The expected number of deaths is obtained by multiplying the rates in the general population by the number of person-years in the exposed group under study.

Age at risk (yr)

	25–34	35–44	45–54	55–64	65–74
Rates in the general population per 1000 person-years	0.933	2.013	0.810	18.774	48.852
Person-years contributed in the exposed group under study	1600y	2000y	1700y	1000y	700y
Number of expected deaths	1.5	4.0	11.6	18.8	34.2

3. By dividing the number of observed deaths ($3 + 8 + 18 + 29 + 51 = 109$) by the number of expected deaths ($1.5 + 4.0 + 11.6 + 18.8 + 34.2 = 70.1$) (and, by convention, multiplying by 100), the ratio of mortalities in the two groups is obtained:

$$\text{SMR} = 100 \times \frac{\text{sum of observed deaths}}{\text{sum of expected deaths}} \quad \frac{109}{70.1} = 155$$

Mortality in the exposed group is 55 per cent higher than for the general population. The comparison is 'age-adjusted' that is, adjusted for any age difference between the workers and the population at large.

Stratification

The process of separating a sample into several subsamples or strata according to specific criteria such as age, socio-economic status, smoking, etc. An example of stratification is shown in the section on standardization (stratification by sex in the glossary). Stratification is often used to control for confounding and to look for interaction (*see* Stratified analysis).

Stratified analysis

Method used to check for confounding or interaction.

Example: a case-control study of lung cancer in a group of railway workers. The information on previous exposure among cases and controls is summarized in a 2 × 2 table.

Exposure to asbestos	Cases	Controls
Yes	58	86
No	30	90
	88	176

$$OR = \frac{58/30}{86/90} = 2.0$$

The exposed worker's risk of developing lung cancer is twice the risk of a non-exposed worker.

If smoking histories among cases and controls are collected, the results can be displayed in a more informative way by stratifying cases and controls according to their smoking status:

Non-smokers

Asbestos exposure	Cases	Controls
Yes	17	38
No	14	44
	31	82

$$OR = \frac{17/14}{38/44} = 1.4$$

Smokers

Asbestos exposure	Cases	Controls
Yes	41	48
No	16	46
	57	94

$$OR = \frac{41/16}{48/46} = 2.5$$

If smoking was the only cause of lung cancer, then the relative risk associated with asbestos would be 1 among smokers as well as non-smokers. This is not the case. Furthermore, the tables show that smoking seems to modify the effect of asbestos exposure. Exposed workers who smoke have a higher relative risk than exposed non-smokers.

Study base

In *cohort studies* the study base is simply the cohort of people exposed and the cohort of people not exposed. In *case-control studies* the population from which the series of cases occur. In *cross-sectional studies* the group of people being studied at that moment in time.

A more comprehensive dictionary of terms can be found in Last (1983).

REFERENCES

Axelson, O. (1978). Aspects of confounding in occupational health epidemiology. *Scandinavian Journal of Work, Environment and Health*, **4**, 85–9.

Last, J. M. (1983). *A dictionary of epidemiology*. Oxford University Press.

Levine, R. J., Symons, M. J., Balogh, S. A., *et al.* (1980). A method for monitoring the fertility of workers: 1. Method and pilot studies. *Journal of Occupational Medicine*, **22**, 781–91.

Lilienfeld, A. M. (1976). *Foundations of epidemiology*. Oxford University Press.

Schilling, R. S. F. (ed.) (1981). *Occupational health practice*. Butterworths, London.

Weeden, R. P. (1989). Were the hatters of New Jersey 'mad'? *American Journal of Industrial Medicine*, **16**, 225–33.

Wegman, D. H. and Peters, J. M. (1974). Polymer fume fever and cigarette smoking. *Annals of Internal Medicine*, **81**, 55–7.

Whorton, D., Krauss, R. M., Marshall, S., and Milby, T. H. (1977). Infertility in male pesticide workers. *Lancet*, **2**, 1259–61.

FURTHER READING

There are a number of other introductory texts that are available for people interested in occupational epidemiology, including the following:

1. Fox, J., Gee, D., Jones, D., and Leon, D. (1982). *Cancer and Work*.

Making sense of workers' experience. City University Statistical Laboratory in collaboration with the Funeral and Municipal Workers' Union, London.

2. Silverstein, M. (1981). *The case of the workplace killers: a manual for cancer detectives on the job*. Published by the International Union, UAW, 8000 E Jefferson, Detroit, Michigan.

3. Jones, D., Smith, P., and Kinnersly, P. (1981). *Radical Statistics Health Group. Two statistical methods for assessing health hazards at work. A guide to occupational cohort studies*. Radical Statistics, London W1V 3DG.

4. Legator, M.S., Harper, B.L., and Scott, M.J. (1985). *The health detective's handbook. A guide to the investigation of environmental health hazards by non-professionals*. The Johns Hopkins University Press, Baltimore and London.

Index

Printed in the United States
By Bookmasters